THE

SHRED

FAT

PROGRAM

BY

ROBERT WILSON

CONTENTS

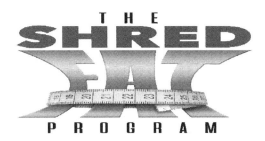

This book is written as a source of information only. The information contained in this book should by no means be considered a substitute for the advice of a qualified medical professional, whom should always be consulted before beginning any new diet, exercise, or other health program.

All efforts have been made to ensure the accuracy of its information, as of the publishing date. All exercises should be carefully studied and clearly understood before attempting them at home or in the gym. The author and the publisher expressly disclaim responsibility for any adverse effects, damages, or losses arising from the use or application of the information contained herein.

For information contact:
Robert Wilson
Website: www.theshredfatprogram.com
Facebook: www.facebook.com/theshredfatprogram

Cover Design: Michael Montes

ACKNOWLEDGMENTS

To Swiss

This book would not exist if not for your words of encouragement and support.

To Michael

Thank you for putting up with my shit. The photographs and the cover are awesome. You have a special talent. It was great to work with you.

To Joan

Thank you for being my fitness model, you're a star. You are an exceptional trainer and your positivity is infectious. I'm happy to have you on my team.

To Deanna and Laura

Thank you for your honest feedback and help. You make living in Saudi easier. I love you both.

To Shred Fat participants

Your hard work and feedback have made this program what it is today. Thank you for trusting in me. There has been blood, sweat and tears, but together we have created a program that is proven to shred fat. The results have been amazing and I'm delighted to have been a positive influence in your life, because most certainly you all have been a positive in mine.

"your time is limited, so don't waste it living someone else's life. Don't be trapped by dogma – which is living with the results of other people's thinking. Don't let the noise of others' opinions drown out your own inner voice. And most important, have the courage to follow your heart and intuition. They somehow already know what you truly want to become. Everything else is secondary".

Steve Jobs

INTRODUCTION

Obesity is a worldwide epidemic! - I have seen first-hand people developing health problems from being obese and the strain it has not only on the individual but on their families too. According to the Irish heart foundation 39% of Irish adults are overweight and 25% are obese. Obese means having excessive body-fat. If you have excessive body fat, you are obese! Once you accept that fact, then you can get to work on doing something about it. We cannot sugarcoat this problem.

The results I have been getting with the Shred Fat Program have been simply amazing. I was encouraged by my clients and friends to put the program into a book and help a larger audience.

Shredding fat is simple, but it is not easy. This program has resulted in fat loss in hundreds of people from around the world. It is an amazing feeling knowing that I have helped so many people lose fat and lead a healthier life.

Traditional weight loss books prescribe a nutrition plan and a training program and send you on your merry way. Although these two components are vital, I have found that people need to be driven and motivated to accomplish any goal; health or otherwise. Which is why the first section of this book is working on your mindset. Without a strong mindset you are destined to fail.

My goal is to help you shred fat, not to make myself sound smart by using scientific words. I have tried as much as possible to make this book easy to read and understand.

This program is not easy, nothing in life worth having is. You have to be committed to see the results. Visit our website and join our Facebook page; interact with others on the same goal as you. Together we are stronger and together we will achieve new heights.

Are you ready?

MINDSET

MINDSET

I will show you what you need to do, but ultimately it is down to how committed are you. I could easily just prescribe the nutrition and exercise plan and leave the rest up to you, but I would be doing you a great disservice. From my years of experience, I find people need to have a strong mindset to accomplish any goal. I will do my best within this section to get you motivated and focused so you can achieve your goal.

On this program you will:

1. Set goals
2. Commit to the program
3. Sort out your sleep patterns
4. Limit your stress levels
5. Create a strong supportive circle of friends
6. Follow the 7-day Reset nutritional plan
7. Follow the subsequent 5-week Shred nutrition plan
8. Do 4 exercise sessions a week

If you fall, then you just have to stand up, dust yourself off and get back on the horse. You need to develop the right mindset to smash your goals. This doesn't come easy; you will be tested. There will be times when you don't want to eat healthy or to go train. But remember that being healthy is not a race, it is a journey; so enjoy the ride.

GOALS ON PAPER

Step one is putting your long term goal on paper. Everyone has different goals, yours might be to look good in the mirror, lose 100 pounds, be a role model for your family or fit into that old bondage outfit that is gathering dust in your wardrobe. Whatever it is, you need to write it down.

Next to your long term goal, put a deadline of when you want to achieve it. This may be a year from now or more. Be ambitious. This program is six weeks long but I hope the information provided will help you make better food choices and lead a healthy active lifestyle for the remainder of your life.

Step two is writing down your short term goal that you will strive to achieve on this 6-week program. You must be specific! - Here are some examples:

- Lose 8 pounds of body fat
- Lose 3 inches off my waist
- Lose two dress sizes
- Fit into my old jeans
- Be able to touch my toes
- Exercise regularly
- Improve strength
- Increase muscles mass
- Be more active with my family

A nice easy approach is proven to be healthier and more enjoyable. If you enjoy it, you will be more likely to stick to it. If you lost 1 inch off your waist every month, after 1 year that would be 12 inches, hell you might need to buy a new bondage costume!

Get some post-it's, write your long term goal on them and stick them around the house to remind you why you're leading a healthier lifestyle, stick that long term goal on the fridge, in the fridge, on your mirror and in your wallet.

Do this now!

THE DREAM BOARD

I like to read entrepreneur books and discuss business ideas, quotes and concepts with my friends. I recently told my girlfriend that I now have twenty things on my list that I will accomplish within the next five years. I got this idea of having a list from Bill Cullen's book "*It's a long way from penny apples*".

My girlfriend said she had something similar and went and showed me her dream board, which was a board in her bedroom with all her dreams on it. It had things she wanted, like having her own business, owning her own house and so on. Can you see her mistake? For one, she calls it a dream. It should be a goal. Dreams rarely come through and having a "dream" board just shows me that: I would like those things, but it will probably never happen.

Where else did she go wrong? Timeline. When does she want to have a business? Is thirty years okay with you, honey? Fancy a house at sixty when the kids have all long gone? No, you take the goal, throw a timeline on that son of a bitch and then you create a plan that will get you there.

How is this all relevant to shredding fat? If you are overweight, you should write down a specific weight you want to be and when you want it by and then you follow a plan in getting there. Simple.

BELIEVE

After writing down your goal, you need to believe that you can achieve it. You have to talk to yourself constantly and convince yourself that you will do it. Don't say "I WANT to lose ten pounds of fat", instead say "I WILL lose ten pounds of fat". The inner dialogue you say to yourself each day makes a massive difference to developing an unbreakable mindset.

Irish mixed martial arts phenomenon Conor Mcgregor said "What you make real in your mind, you eventually make real in your life". Conor told himself he will be the world champion, actually, Conor told the whole world he will become world champion. He visualized himself everyday lifting that belt, not achieving his goal didn't even come into his frame of mind. A solid determined mindset with support from close friends can bring your goals to fruition. Conor grinded day in and day out for ten years. He had many failures and set-backs but he never lost sight of his goal and became UFC world featherweight champion.

Each morning I want you to wake up and repeat that long term goal to yourself, say it out loud and say it before you go to bed. Eat, sleep and breath your long term goal.

VISUALIZE

Everybody should meditate each day. Not only is it relaxing, but it gives you a sense of clarity around what is important in your life. I suggest you lie down for ten minutes a day in a quiet room and visualize yourself achieving your goal. Focus on the emotions that you feel having accomplished it. See yourself being happy that all your hard work has paid off. You have ignored instant gratification along the road and that the fruits of your labor are everything you imagined.

You need to tap into your subconscious mind and change your thought process. The thoughts you have about yourself might be holding you back, it will take a lot of work to rewire your brain to making you believe you can do whatever you want. Visualizing is challenging at first, but just keep working on seeing yourself achieving, it will burn a fire inside your mind which will be needed when times get tough.

Create a positive internal dialogue and tell yourself that you WILL accomplish your goal and that failure is not even an option. Speak about yourself positively and let no negative thoughts or emotions fester for long.

When I find myself procrastinating, I close my eyes and see myself achieving my goal for 10 seconds. Then open my eyes and get to work. It's the only way I refrained from Facebook stalking while writing this book.

ACTION

Your goals should now be written down and you have begun the process of believing in yourself. Now it's time for action. You have got to put the work in because there is no quick fix or magic pill. It's hard work and determination each and every day. There is blood, sweat and tears with sacrifices and heart aches thrown in. The information in this book must be applied over and over again.

As Apollo Creed told Rocky "There is no tomorrow", Read that quote again, and for a third time, actually say it out loud. Today is the day to start, not Monday or after your vacation in three weeks, or when the kids are back in school. That mindset is for the people who hit the snooze button and who post I hate Monday pictures on Instagram. There will always be an excuse not to start, the time to start is right now.

INSTANT GRATIFICATION

Being committed to the program and working on it day in and day out is the hardest thing of all. You have got to constantly keep on this program especially when times get hard and you don't feel like it. You have to keep repeating your long term goal to yourself so you can stay focused.

Instant gratification will distract you from your goal. Most people want everything now and are not willing to work hard for it. Sitting at home watching Game of Thrones is a lot easier than hitting the gym. Ordering takeout is a lot easier than cooking. But watching all seven seasons of Game of Thrones shouldn't be written on your fridge, if it is you have a problem. You have to sacrifice what you want now to achieve what you want most. I repeat: you have to sacrifice what you want now to achieve what you want most.

PATIENCE AND PERSEVERANCE

The road to your goal is not an empty highway with the wind in your hair and Free Bird on the radio. Nope, it's a congested road at rush hour and you're hitting every red light. Horns are beeping and you feel like telling the person who just cut you off to go fuck themselves. If you have lived in Jeddah, Saudi Arabia, this is a normal day while driving.

You could do a U-turn at any time and be watching Jon Snow protect a wall with your feet up and a Snickers ice cream in hand. Sadly, most people take this U-turn not realizing that the traffic will subside. Every mile is progress and anything of value is not going to be easy. So take a deep breath, remain calm, move slowly through the traffic and don't pay attention to the driver who cut you off. Do these things, and you will get to your destination.

ENVIRONMENT

You are a product of your environment. Jim Rohn said "you are the average of the five people you spend the most time with". If your five people are lazy, unproductive people than most likely your life will follow the same path. On the other hand, if you are surrounded by five healthy, motivated people most likely you will become healthy and motivated too.

My circle of five are all positive, healthy, enthusiastic and successful people; we breed off each other's successes. My friend's successes are mine and vice a versa. We help push each other because we are on the same road. We haven't always been this way, but with a change in mindset from one or two we can bring the circle to new heights.

To be healthy and to reach your goals you need to have people around you to push you when you don't feel like it. If your circle like takeaways each night and binge drinking every weekend most likely that is what you will be doing too. You may manage to be healthy for a few weeks or months but ultimately that circle will pull you back into their way of thinking. You WILL fail and go back to your old ways.

If you are in a bad spot and you don't have positive people in your life, then join a health club, a sport or social club. Trust me, surrounding yourself with like-minded people will lead you on the same path. Surround yourself with people you think are better than you and that will raise you up. Fake it until you make it if you must.

My advice which is never easy to hear is to get rid of the friends, girlfriends, boyfriends, spouses or anybody who doesn't support your goal or have your back no matter what. They are energy vampires who only want to bring you down to their level. These people will make fun of your goal and will be jealous of your success. They will call you crazy and will try guilt tripping you into their way off thinking. Fuck these people.

MOTIVATION

I'm addicted to following and learning anything I can from successful people that come from all walks of life. Steve Jobs, Alan Sugar, Dame Dash, Gary Vaynerchuk and Will Smith are examples of men who done everything in their power to be at the top of their game. I read constantly to take inspiration from successful people. They had a goal, made a plan and put their head down until they got to where they wanted to be.

I send my circle inspirational quotes and videos every damn day. It fires me up listening to successful people. If it fires me up, I send it to my circle to get them fired up. In return they send me things similar. What are we doing? We are creating a positive environment within our circle. We might all have different goals but by motivating each other it pushes us to work hard for them.

Follow successful people, read quotes, read books, watch lectures and motivational videos, listen to speeches and podcasts. Everyday find ways to get the fire burning inside you, especially during times of procrastination. Take inspirational quotes and put them around your house, around your office, hell even tattoo them on your arm if it gets you fired up.

There were days where I didn't want to sit down and write this book, but I get daily messages from my friends and it gets me back writing. We all feel like not doing things but the beautiful thing about having a strong circle is they will be your crutches when you need them most.

MY BROTHER

My brother Luke failed his leaving certificate (final second-level exams) miserably. So badly he didn't want to share his results with anyone. He didn't work hard and was easily distracted with having fun, which is common with young teens from the area where we grew up. I was employed in Saudi Arabia at the time, so I made it a mission of mine to get him motivated. After some time, I got him motivated enough to get a personal training qualification just like I did but fitness just wasn't for him.

After sometime passed that course built a fire within him to make something of himself, so he decided to do his leaving certificate again. Being so determined to get good grades, he made himself accountable and posted his old leaving certificate results on his Facebook for all friends and family to see. Now he had to put the work in. Luke got a whopping 400 points in his leaving certificate and is now in Maynooth University studying business and finance.

Change your mindset, change your life.

YOUR PAST DOESN'T DEFINE YOU

The past is gone; the universe doesn't give a shit about who you were. Your past mistakes and failures are irrelevant. When I was younger I was a fucking demon. I used to get into trouble, take drugs, drink excessively and I'm sure some people from my past would have bad things to say about me. But I can't dwell on that, I'm this person today and I can't relate to the person I once was. The late great Mohammad Ali said "The man who views the world at 50 the same as he did at 20 has wasted 30 years of his life".

So take responsibility that you have let yourself go a little and from today become a better version of yourself. Don't let people's opinions affect how you perceive yourself. You are fucking awesome, believe that and forget the past, live in the present and visualize your future.

INTEREST/COMMITMENT

Interest is reading this book, commitment is reading it over and over and applying the information day in and day out. Interest is saying you will start on Monday, commitment is throwing out all the crap in your fridge now and making your new shopping list. Interested is looking up exercise workouts, commitment is lacing up and going to the gym.

Everybody wants to be healthy, but not everybody is willing to work for it. Everybody wants the prize, but not everybody is willing to pay the price. Everybody will share an inspirational quote, but not everybody will follow the advice. Are you interested or committed?

PLACE THE BLAME

The only person to blame for you being unhealthy is yourself. The only person to blame for you not being happy is yourself. The only person to blame for being stuck in a rut is yourself. It's not the governments fault, it's not your ex-spouses fault and it's not your jobs fault. It's your fault. Harsh? I couldn't care less. To excel at leading a healthy happy life you need to understand that all the emotions you feel are created by yourself. You're responsible for your own happiness and health. You and you alone.

Blame yourself for being fat, blame yourself for being lazy and blame yourself if you're unhappy. Once you place the blame on yourself and take responsibility for your health and happiness, then you can build the foundation necessary to get up and take control.

START WINNING

You need to start off the day on the right foot. Which means putting your feet on the floor when your alarm goes off. Do not hit the snooze button. If you hit the snooze button, you are mentally weak. Why did you set the alarm at that time in the first place? Last night you set a wake up time and were determined to get up but this morning you would rather five more minutes' sleep.

Nobody likes getting out of bed when the alarm rings, nobody. The alarm going off is your first challenge of the day, are you going to fall at the first hurdle?

I'm a 5 AM guy, but I wasn't always. I just trained myself daily to throw my feet out of the bed when the alarm rings. I say my goal out loud, which at this time is to finish this book. I refuse to be mentally weak, especially in the first few waking seconds.

Get in the zone and no more snooze button.

SHREDDING FAT IS SIMPLE

This can't be true right? 65% of people in Ireland are obese. If it was simple, then nobody would be overweight right? It is simple but that's not to be confused with easy.

Shredding fat is simple, because after reading this book you will have a proven process to achieve your goal. You must be mentally in the game, motivated and determined. A nutrition plan and an exercise plan which most books provide are useless unless the individual accessing them is motivated and focused to do the work. How can you follow a plan when you are not getting enough sleep or your surrounded by negative people?

Let's be honest here, I don't know who you are. You might want to lose 5lbs or 300lbs. You might just want to eat healthier and live a better life. You might be a vegetarian and can't follow some parts of the program. You might have chronic back pain, arthritis or recovering from knee surgery. So, understand there is no one size fits all program. Although this program will cater to most. You might have to edit the exercise and nutrition plan to cater to your needs.

WHY CAN'T YOU KEEP IT SIMPLE?

A lack of motivation and hard-work are the culprits. Many folks start off with good intentions but after a few weeks or when life gets a little bit hectic they end up packing it in. It's easy to be motivated at the beginning, but when life throws a few curveballs your way then motivation goes out the window.

There is never an excuse not to eat properly and to sneak in an exercise session once or twice a week. You may have a busy lifestyle but I can guarantee you there are people who have a busier schedule than you and are getting work done.

To achieve my goal of writing this book I refrained from watching any TV or films. I do a 48-hour work-week, do ten hours personal training and coaching, study for my leadership and management course, work on my other business endeavors, spend time with my daughter, workout and write my book. As I said before you have to sacrifice what you want now for what you want most.

If you watch boxsets on a regular basis and have time to sit and watch Soccer Saturday or any of the soaps, you're not that busy. You have time to exercise and prepare meals. You're just making excuses. Bill Cullen, Ireland's self-made millionaire works 16 hours a day and still manages a workout at 6am each morning. You can make all the excuses you want. Everyone has the same 24 hours in each day. You, me and Bill Cullen, what you choose to do each day is what defines you.

Health is a journey, it's not a race. I want you to enjoy it so of course watch some TV and films but only do these things if you're making progress towards your goal. Same with eating junk food, ask yourself do you deserve it? If you did, then hell yeah open a bottle of wine and order a pizza.

SLEEP

We mentioned earlier no snooze button, that's a rule and you can't break it. You must start the day on the right path. You should aim for between six to eight hours of sleep each night. We would all love to go to bed at the same time each and every night and wake up at the same time each morning, this is not always feasible, but try your best to have a good sleep routine. I work best when I sleep at 10 PM and wake at 5 AM, I'm really productive in the mornings and love getting lots of work done while people sleep. People don't start calling me or emailing me until 8 AM so I get over two hours of solid work done before people even wake up. But that's me, you need to find the balance for you.

A lack of sleep slows down your metabolism to conserve energy which is not what we want. The hormone cortisol is released which increases your appetite and puts your body in a catabolic state. A catabolic state is simply a breakdown of muscle tissues. When you sleep I want your body in an anabolic state. In an anabolic state your body will repair muscle tissue and increase your metabolic rate. Without good sleep you will not get the most out of this program.

People who sleep less generally eat more. I want you to view sleep as your body getting serviced each night. Your metabolism needs to be firing on all cylinders to maximize your ability to shred fat. I don't know your work schedule or lifestyle so make your own sleep routine where you get the required hours. During sleep you will burn fat and your body will build muscle, sleep is the time when your body repairs itself. If your sleep is not in order you won't want to work out and you won't be productive throughout the day.

If you are having trouble sleeping here are some tips

- Sleep at the same time each night.
- Cut out caffeine after 4pm.
- Don't watch any TV two hours before sleep.
- Don't look at your phone screen two hours before sleep.
- Read before sleeping.
- Light candles instead of room lights.
- Exercise daily.
- Warm bath at night.
- Drink chamomile tea at night.
- Keep a clean bedroom with clean sheets.
- Find a new job if necessary.

LIMIT STRESS

With today's lifestyle it is hard not to be stressed. The Irish economy went through many years of hardship which is why I moved abroad, but don't let these situations affect your health. You just have to limit your daily stress levels because just like sleep, being stressed decreases metabolism and increases the hormone cortisol.

If you work too many hours, have family issues, suffer from depression or all three put together then please look after yourself and address these issues. I know it's easier said than done. Eating healthy and exercising can help relieve some off your stress so do lead a healthy lifestyle. After I exercise I have no negative energy, all my energy is wasted in the gym.

I don't want you to just look good, I want you to feel good and be the best person you can be for you and your family. Get your life in balance and remove any negative people, cut down work hours if necessary and surround yourself with like-minded positive people.

Summary

- Set short term and long term goals.
- Your long term goal should be repeated each morning before you get out of bed and before you sleep. Post it in as many places as you like.
- Short term goals should be set every 4-6 weeks.
- Have goals with deadlines and follow a set plan for getting there.
- Use positive words and create a positive internal dialogue with yourself.
- Believe in yourself and visualize yourself achieving your long term goal.
- You WILL achieve your goal!
- Act on your goal immediately. There is no tomorrow. The time is right now.
- Persistence separates the strong from the weak.
- Instant gratification will distract you from long term success, other people want everything now and are not willing to work hard for it. You are not other people.
- You have to sacrifice what you want now to achieve what you want most.
- Have patience and persevere. Times will get tough and you will lack morale and motivation. It's meant to be hard, but these hardships make achieving your goal all the more worthwhile. The sweet is never as sweet without the sour.
- Make your environment positive and supporting. You are the average of the five people you spend the most time with. Choose wisely.
- Find daily motivation and share with your circle and get them to do the same.
- Your past doesn't define you. You are a new person from today. Never forget where you came from, but know exactly where you are going.
- Be committed and apply all the advice in this book with your full dedication and enthusiasm.
- Interest is just reading this book, commitment is applying it day in and day out.
- Take responsibility for where you are in life right now and stop blaming others. Then and only then can you start moving forward. That long term goal is yours for the taking. You and you alone are held accountable if you don't achieve it.
- Start your day of right and don't hit the snooze button.
- Shredding fat is simple, not to be confused with easy.
- Only watch TV if your life is in balance. Don't let TV get in the way of exercise, good food or sleep. Use it as a reward only.
- Get six to eight hours of sleep a night. Change your lifestyle if you struggle with this.
- Limit the stress in your life. Stress decreases your metabolic rate and morale. It's impossible to avoid but making small changes to your lifestyle or cutting people out of your life make a massive difference.

NUTRITION

NUTRITION

You should already have your goals down on paper and be adjusting your sleeping pattern. In this section I shouldn't have to teach you that a kale shake is healthier than a donut, but I will explain my reasoning (without getting to nerdy) behind the shred fat nutrition plan.

On week one you will follow the Reset Nutrition Plan which was carefully created to give you high quality nutrients without taxing your digestive system. Then for the remaining five weeks you will follow the Shred Nutrition Plan which lets you choose the foods you like from the lists I provide at the end of this section. On the Shred Nutrition Plan I'm not going to make you eat fish if you don't like it. I'm not going to make you have a breakfast if you don't like eating first thing in the morning. I'm allowing you to build your own food plan, so if you don't like a certain food, then simply don't eat it. A nutrition plan with foods you enjoy will be more enjoyable and sustainable long term.

SHRED FAT

The goal of this program is to shred fat while trying to maintain as much muscle mass as possible. I'm putting in a lot of effort to write this book because a lot of weight loss programs just focus on losing weight, not caring where the weight comes from. These programs are based purely on the weighing scales. There is only one type of weight I want you to lose and that is FAT. The visceral body fat that has no business being on your frame.

Traditional weight loss programs do generally make people lose "weight". But when they lose the weight and look in the mirror, they don't see much of a difference. They will just see a slightly smaller version of themselves. They don't see much definition in their mid-section or look at all athletic like the person on the book cover. This can be de-moralizing; how can you remain motivated without visual results? How can you stick to a program if you are not getting positive feedback for your sacrifices and hard-work?

On the Shred Fat Program, you will lose fat and build muscle. I want my clients and anyone following this program to be the first to take off their t-shirts when the sun comes out, or even take them off when it's cold because you have that much confidence in your physique.

DO NOT CALORIE RESTRICT LONG TERM

The Reset Nutrition Plan on this program is calorie restricting but it is only for seven days. It's essential to get your digestive system running smoothly, encourage a healthy internal ecosystem and to give your digestive organs a break from all the damage you have been doing to it over the years.

Calorie restricting over the long term, which many tend to do can be detrimental to your health. I suggest no longer than seven days every two or three months. Here are a few side-effects of restricting calories long term:

- Slows down your metabolism
- Loss of strength
- Loss of muscle mass
- Disrupts your endocrine system
- Increased depression
- Decrease in energy levels
- Decreased sex drive

Our bodies are not made to have calorie deficits for long periods of time so do not Reset for longer than seven days. Life is hard enough with work, studying, family and exercising and on top of all that you want to eat a calorie restricting diet? Fuck that, I'm eating often, and you're going to do the same.

FOLLOW LOGIC

Not only do traditional programs want you to eat less, they want you to exercise more. If I'm eating a small amount of calories every day and you want me to go exercise, trust me I'm not showing up. You won't have the energy or drive to do it well anyway, especially if you haven't exercised in a long time and you've been on the "eat everything diet".

On week one while following the Reset nutrition plan, I just want you to focus on getting quality sleep, balancing your lifestyle environment and following the nutrition plan to a tee. Exercise is a stress to the body, so take it easy these seven days and just be as active as you possibly can. This can be very challenging for those of you who are used to eating a lot of processed foods and soda. Your body will be craving sugar so just load up on vegetables and lean meats; these you can eat in abundance and don't worry about exercising until the reset phase is over. For others, you may be able to start the workouts during the reset phase, but start light and focus on the proper exercise technique. Listen to your body and enjoy the journey.

I will say it again: please take it easy during your seven-day Reset. Only add strenuous exercise after it. We are building a solid foundation during these seven days. This doesn't mean be inactive. Do light activities like walking, swimming, yoga or cycling; Just move and move often.

METABOLISM

A little science behind the shred fat process, so bear with me. Shredding fat is all about increasing your metabolism. I don't want to get too scientific because I want you to enjoy this book. I could easily use big words that make me sound smart but I'm a Dublin boy and I want to keep it simple. Most importantly I need you to understand what your metabolism is and how it works. The main component of fat loss is knowing the ways to manipulate your metabolism. Once you have this knowledge you will make better health choices in the future.

Your metabolism is how fast your body burns calories to convert to energy. Now that's a simplification, and doesn't tell the whole story but it's all you need to know. Google metabolism if you want to learn more, but we're not here to learn about the chemical processes inside living cells, we're here to shred fat.

The 4 ways of calorie expenditure:

1. Resting Metabolic Rate (RMR) equates to between 60-75% of total calorie expenditure in the body, it is how many calories your body burns when at complete rest. RMR takes up the majority of the calories that you eat on a daily basis. On the Shred Fat Program, we are looking to maintain or increase muscle mass, the more muscle mass you have the higher your RMR. So a good weight lifting program is a must to shred fat.
2. Physical Activity Level (PAL) equates to between 15-30% of total calorie expenditure in the body. Your PAL is any movement you do daily, the more active you are, the more calories you will burn. Just don't expect to burn many calories by reaching for the remote control and shovelling bacon cheese fries into your mouth. The Shred Fat Program incorporates some of the best fat burning exercises you can do to increase PAL.
3. Thermic Effect of Feeding (TEF) equates to between 5 to 15% of total calorie expenditure in the body. It is how many calories you burn digesting food. The Shred Fat nutrition plan encourages you to eat many times a day. Eating five times each day will increase the calories you burn while digesting, isn't that great news.
4. Non-Exercise Activity Thermogenesis (NEAT) equates to about 5% of total calorie expenditure. It is something you cannot change and is written already in your genetic makeup. Luckily this only accounts for a small percentage of calorie expenditure. You can't pick your parents, so nothing I can do for you here.

Increasing your BMR, PAL and TEF are the core of the Shred Fat Program.

NUTRITION PLANNING

A solid nutrition plan is vital; without it you will not reach your goal. You must follow the Reset nutrition plan and the subsequent Shred nutrition plan as religiously as possible. I like to see the nutrition plan as a game of chess. The chess pieces are the foods you can eat; so choose wisely.

The Reset is your starting game, its preparing your pieces for the battle. It's getting your pieces into advantageous positions from the get go. With a poor starting game you will find it difficult in getting into positions to start attacking the king (your goal). The Reset phase is vital because it prepares your body for the exercise program that starts in week two. It gets you in the zone mentally and physically.

The Shred phase is the middle game, you should deliberate what pieces to move and at what times. You have to use your intelligence. Mistakes are expected when starting out, but learning from these mistakes will make you a better chess player. You will select which foods you like from the lists provided and you will time your complex carbohydrate meal around your workouts.

The end game is when the king is in sight and you want that checkmate. There are many different ways of getting it. Eat the foods that you enjoy from the lists and just keep at it day in and day out. Once you achieve checkmate, reset the pieces and play again.

THE SHRED FAT RESET PHASE

Say good bye to the junk food and sodas, they are killing you from the inside. Consuming those foods and drinks damage your endothelial cells (thin layer of cells than line the interior surface of blood vessels). Plaque forms in these cells which restrict blood flow to your organs and this plaque causes inflammation of the cell walls.

Heart disease is the number one killer in Ireland, killing ten thousand people a year, this equates to 33% of total deaths in Ireland. This is a scary statistic; a significant proportion of this figure can be avoided if people just made better health choices.

A nutrition plan based on fruit, vegetables, lean meats and healthy fats helps heal these endothelial cells and will remove plaque, lower cholesterol and improve blood flow. This massively reduces your risk of heart attacks, or do you still want that heart bypass surgery for Christmas?

The Reset phase is eating clean natural foods with limited complex carbohydrates for seven days. This will reduce bloating and will give your digestive system a break from all the bad food and drink you have been shovelling into it. Your body already helps breakdown substances and attempts to cleanse your body daily. When resetting you're giving your digestive system a break and in return promoting a healthy internal ecosystem. You will feel like a new you after seven days, and will notice a difference on the scale and on your waist.

The Shred Fat Reset Phase will include the following:

- Fruits
- Vegetables
- Lean meats
- Nuts and seeds
- Grass fed butter
- Aloe Vera
- Green Tea
- Coffee/ Black tea
- Herbs and spices
- Balsamic vinegar
- Olive oil
- Sea salt
- Fish oil
- Multi-vitamin and mineral

See the Reset plan at end of this section

AFTER THE RESET

Once your seven-day Reset is complete you are straight into the Shred Phase. The Shred Phase is a five-week nutrition plan and is based around lots of vegetables, lean meats, and healthy fats which will strengthen your immune system and make you feel like a beast. You can, however, have complex carbohydrates like sweet potato and brown rice, but these can only be consumed after your training sessions.

If you train late at night, then you can save that carbohydrate rich meal for breakfast the next morning. Which is what a lot of people do for they love the Oatmeal Bowl (in recipe section) for breakfast. Make the nutrition plan your own, but try to stick to the list as much as possible.

For you vegetarians: you can add soy, beans and legumes to the list. But, for everybody that eats meat and eggs, then I advise to stick to the list. Make a shopping list from the food lists at the end of this section. Stick to your shopping list! If it's not on the list, then don't buy it. I repeat: If it's not on the list then don't buy it.

EAT FREQUENTLY

In the Shred phase, you will be eating five times a day instead of the usual three square meals a day. By eating five times a day you will increase your Thermic Effect of Feeding (TEF). This means you will burn more calories a day because your body has to work to digest food five times daily. Your digestive system will always be on the go throughout the day. The meals are smaller portions so you will be less bloated (which alone takes inches off your waist) and your digestive system doesn't have to work too hard because the foods you are eating are of the highest quality and are easily digestible.

WATER

I want you drinking at least two litres of water each day. Water will:

- help your digestion system work efficiently
- keep muscles hydrated
- helps the transportation of nutrients
- slow down the absorption rate making you feel fuller for longer

Make sure you drink enough water each day and drink water in the gym before, during and after your workouts. You have to replace the lost fluids from sweating. Stick to water only, no energy drinks!

One litre of your recommended water intake will be the following homemade drink. Take a litre of warm water and squeeze in half a lemon and add a pinch of sea salt. Now you have one of the healthiest drinks known to man. This drink is a must in the Reset phase, then it is optional in the Shred Phase.

Benefits of this drink:

- Reduced blood sugar levels
- Increased energy levels
- Anti-inflammatory
- Immune system booster
- Alkalizing in the body
- Regulates metabolism
- Fat loss

GREENS

You will eat lots of green vegetables; they are super packed with nutrients. Leafy green vegetables in particular because they have more nutrition per calorie than any other food. Your plate will be mostly green and you can eat as much as you want because they are:

- Low in calories
- Low in fat
- Full of antioxidants
- High in fibre
- High in iron
- High in calcium

There are over a thousand edible green leaves and vegetables you can eat, pick and choose the ones you prefer. Wash all vegetables with a vegetable wash or with lemon water.

Greens to eat:

- Kale
- Collards
- Spinach
- Bok Choi
- Broccoli
- Cabbage
- Artichoke
- Asparagus
- Sprouts
- Chives
- Rocket
- Romaine Lettuce

VEGETABLES

In the Reset phase you won't be eating grains or potatoes so you will need to load up on some root vegetables because they are full of fibre and filled with slow burning carbohydrates which is just what you need.

During Reset load up on these root vegetables:

- Carrots

- Turnips
- Beets
- Parsnips

Once the Shred Phase starts you can add sweet potatoes, which is also a root vegetable. Root vegetables are your main complex carbohydrates on this program. They are nutrient dense and will help regulate glucose levels and will help you feel fuller for longer for they stay in the digestive tract.

Also, add in these vegetables to give your body a wide range of nutrients.

- Peppers
- Onions
- Eggplant
- Tomatoes
- Mushrooms

It amazes me that the majority of people in the world don't eat green vegetables every day. My parents always shouted at me: "Eat your greens". My Dad worked as a Greengrocer when I was young and he didn't make too much money, so most of our food was vegetables and fruit. At the time I wanted pizza and chips like other kids on the street, but I was very fortunate that my family couldn't afford those items as it kept us all healthy. It can be a challenge today because there is so much processed food and all extremely cheap, but instil good eating habits in your house hold or health problems may come knocking.

Steamed vegetables are better than boiled and note that the longer you cook your vegetables the more nutrients they lose.

PROTEIN

You must eat protein at every meal. This macronutrient will help speed up your metabolism, build muscle and will increase fat burning. Protein will make you feel fuller for longer. Protein mostly gets broken down in the stomach, other macro nutrients like carbohydrates and fats get broken down in the intestines. All food increases your bodies TEF, but protein gives your body an even higher metabolic boost, even higher than carbohydrates or fats!

On the Shred Fat Program, you will eat a lot of quality protein because the problem with most diets is that clients feel hungry and it's hard to stay committed to a nutrition plan when you're getting hunger pangs. You don't need to calorie count, just have a good portion of protein at each meal.

Eat approximately 30 grams of protein per meal, that's a 4-ounce chicken, steak or fish. If you weigh more and feel hungry then add an extra 1-2 ounces. Remember we're trying to maintain or build muscle too.

When cooking meat stick to grilled, boiled or baked as much as possible. If frying (because who doesn't like a fried steak) use coconut oil only. It can withstand high temperatures and is a healthy alternative to vegetable oils.

Proteins to eat:

- Fish
- Chicken
- Turkey
- Protein powder
- Lean red meat
- Liver
- Eggs
- Lean pork

EAT FATS

I want you eating fats and plenty of them. Fat is a macronutrient just like carbohydrates and protein and is vital, yes, vital for your body to work efficiently.

Monounsaturated fats are found in red meat, avocados, nuts and olive oil. Polyunsaturated fats are found in nuts, seeds, fish and leafy greens. These fats should be consumed every day, because they are easily digestible.

Polyunsaturated fats include omega 3 and omega 6. These are both essential fatty acids that your body needs. They lower bad cholesterol, reduce high blood pressure, increase metabolism, make stronger joints and improve brain function. It is hard to get enough of these fats daily which is why you will also supplement with fish oil.

Avoid trans fats and for the most part saturated fats. Coconut oil and grass-fed butter are the exception to the no saturated fat rule. They are superfoods that will help your immune system, increase muscle growth and repair. These should still be taken in moderation, so don't be chewing on a block of butter.

Fats you will consume:

- Fish
- Nuts
- Avocados
- Olive oil
- Seeds
- Coconut oil
- Grass-fed butter

CARBOHYDRATES

Carbohydrates are the most important source of energy for the body. They can be found in grains, fruits, vegetables and dairy products. Your digestive system converts these carbohydrates to glucose (blood sugar). Your body uses this glucose for energy in cells, tissues and organs.

There are two types of Carbohydrates: Simple and Complex. Simple Carbohydrates include sugars found in fruits, vegetables and dairy products and also refined sugars. Complex Carbohydrates include grains, breads and starchy vegetables.

The number one complex carbohydrate for you to eat after your workouts is sweet potato. It is full of anti-oxidant nutrients, anti-inflammatory properties, fibre, and is great at regulating blood sugar levels. I recommend that this be the main carbohydrate in your post workout meal. Steam it, boil it or cut into French fries and grill it. There are many ways to prepare this amazing food.

Stay away from all types of bread, they are all highly processed. Brown rice is fine a couple of times a week, I even added white rice for people because again this program has to cater for the individual. My Filipino friends here in Saudi, have white rice with every meal. Telling them not to eat white rice is like telling Father Dougal McGuire not to hit the red button. Eat rice in moderation and choose the other complex carbohydrates if possible.

The complex carbohydrates you can only have after a workout are:

- Sweet potato
- Quinoa
- Oats
- Hulled barley
- Brown rice-sparingly
- White rice- sparingly

Portion size for all carbohydrates listed above should be no bigger than your fist.

FOOD TIMINGS

Eating the right foods at the right times is by far the best way to shred fat. In the Shred Phase you are able to eat certain carbohydrates after your workouts. I'm going to throw a little scientific mumbo jumbo in here because I find it's important for you to know why.

Your liver takes the brunt for all that alcohol you drink and is the sweet spot for boxers to target when looking for body shots, but it is also a storage unit for glycogen (stored energy). The liver helps maintain optimal blood glucose (sugar) levels. When the liver is full of glycogen the body is said to be in an anabolic state, this means your body is building as opposed to breaking down. This is the state you need to be in to build muscle and recover from your workouts. So eating a carbohydrate meal after working out will replenish your glycogen levels and not be stored as excess fat.

Insulin is secreted from the pancreas into your bloodstream when blood glucose increases. Insulin helps glucose to be stored in the liver, muscle and fat cells. Insulin's number one job is to control blood glucose levels. The higher your blood glucose levels, the higher amounts of insulin are released. If your blood glucose levels are always high, then you have no chance of burning that excess fat and you increase your risk of the ever popular diabetes. So on this program I prescribe only to eat certain carbohydrates after a workout. To keep you in a fat burning state and to balance your blood glucose levels.

The hormone glucagon does the opposite job insulin does. When blood glucose is low, glucagon is released from the liver to bring blood glucose levels back to normal. To maximize fat shredding, your blood glucose levels should be balanced. After a workout, blood glucose levels and stored glycogen will be low. So when you eat your carbohydrate meal after working out, your blood glucose levels won't spike because the glucose will be stored in the muscle and liver; not as visceral fat. Result!

This carbohydrate meal is what we call a re-feed in the fitness industry, you are just topping up with sugars to be stored for energy to be used later. So after each workout you can add certain carbohydrates to your meal, which makes me workout more because I love sweet potato fries.

FOOD SHOPPING

I recommend that you only go food shopping on a full stomach. This will make you less impulsive, and the cheese cake won't find its way into your basket. If the cheese cake is not in your fridge, then you won't be able to eat it.

If you recognise that you can't trust yourself to shop alone, then go shopping with one of your circle and they will keep you on the right path. This is all mental warfare; we all want to eat shit food. Sugar is very addictive, especially when we are hungry and we see them beautiful glistening wrappers and can only imagine what they will taste like. Kick temptation in the teeth, you're on a mission!

I have a tendency to check in on my clients regularly and look in their fridges and cupboards. I was so in demand in Saudi I could afford to threaten clients that if I caught them cheating that I wouldn't train them anymore. I don't like wasting my time, I only train people who are 100% committed to getting to where they want to be. Who knows, I might knock on your door and have a look in your fridge. I'm from Dublin so I can pick a lock... joking!

READ THE LABELS

Make this a habit on everything you buy in the grocery store. It will help you make healthy decisions to keep you on the straight and narrow. The food you consume should have as little ingredients as possible. Basically if there are more than a couple of ingredients in a product or you don't recognise some of the ingredients then don't eat it. Rice is rice and fish is fish; it's as simple as that. A good tip is to shop only the perimeter of a supermarket, usually the processed food is in the middle aisles.

Sugar in our food is a massive problem and the food industries are smart at hiding sugars. Refrain from eating anything with:

- Glucose
- Fructose
- High glucose corn syrup
- Sucrose
- Barley Malt
- Malt Syrup
- Dextrose
- Maltose.

Beware of companies advertising Sugar Free, Fat Free and even Organic. Always read the label and you will see what it is you are putting in your body. For example, Organic products to be able to be called Organic only need one item to be organic in that product, the rest can be the sugars and other nasty processed shit that's bad for your health. It's all just a trick to make you think you're making a healthy choice.

You can't go wrong with reading the label or by just buying fresh fruit, vegetables, rice, lean meats, nuts and seeds. These have no labels at all.

SUPPLEMENTS

There are some supplements I want you to take on this program to optimize your health. It is hard to get adequate amounts of some nutrients each day so take these 4 supplements:

- **Aloe Vera Gel**-This must be taken over the 6 weeks of the program. Aloe Vera aids in digestion. It is favoured by those looking to maintain a healthy digestive system and a natural energy level. Take 100ml each morning upon waking, I don't know of a better way to start the day. I recommend Forever Aloe Vera gel, for it's the closest to the real thing as you can get.
- **Fish Oil**- It's very difficult to get enough healthy fats from diet alone. Supplementing with fish oil will increase your intake of healthy fats like Omega 3 and 6. Take 2 capsules twice a day of fish oil that come from sardines, salmon and anchovies. It does the business at shredding fat, decreasing inflammation and improves brain function.
- **Multi-Vitamin and Mineral** tablets (MVM's)- It is very difficult to get all the vitamins and minerals you need from food alone, taking MVM's gives you extra vitamins and minerals that your diet might be lacking otherwise. Taking a serving first thing in the morning gives your body essential vitamins and minerals to kick-start your day, for me there is no better breakfast than supplying your body with good nutrients and supplements. It sets you off on the right path. Make taking your MVM's first thing in the morning a daily ritual.
- **Protein Powder**- I suggest getting a plant based protein, Garden of Life sell an amazing product. If cost is an issue you may buy whey protein, but only take if you can tolerate dairy products. I know I said no processed food, but protein powder is the only exception. Protein shakes are big for a reason; they are super convenient and easy to digest. You can take one after your workout or when you haven't got time for a meal, it will keep your body in an anabolic state. Without a regular intake of protein your body will burn muscle for energy which will decrease your metabolic rate.

THE 7-DAY RESET PLAN

Wake up and be confident that following the Reset plan will be a walk in the park. Have meals prepared the day before you start if you're a busy bee. No bad food should be in your cupboards and your circle of friends are behind you. This is the beginning of a new you.

- You cannot drink bottled fruit juices or sodas.

- You cannot eat processed food.
- You cannot eat fast foods or sweets.
- You cannot eat refined carbohydrates like rice, pasta or bread.
- No potatoes or anything with flour.

You can drink two Coffees or black tea a day in the Reset Phase. Coffee and tea is where most of us get our antioxidants, so cutting it out is plain silly. Try not adding any milk or dairy if possible and use stevia to sweeten if needs be.

Eat every 2-3 hours to keep your metabolism firing on all cylinders

Upon Waking
Drink 100ml of Aloe Vera Gel and a glass of water
Prepare a litre of warm water with half a fresh squeezed lemon and a pinch of sea salt. To sweeten you can add a small amount of organic honey. Drink this throughout the day.

Meal one (minimum 10 minutes after drinking your Aloe Vera)
1-2 eggs- boiled, poached, scrambled or in an omelette
Cucumber and carrots. Eat raw or simply juice them.
2 Fish oil capsules and a multi-vitamin and mineral

Snack one
An apple

Meal Two
A large multi-coloured salad with grilled/oven chicken or fish. (Olive oil, balsamic vinegar and lemon juice are the only dressings you can use).
Snack two
6- 8 almonds (cucumbers, carrots optional)
Meal Three
Grilled/oven chicken or fish with mixed vegetables (choose from vegetable list in Shred Phase)

THE 5-WEEK NUTRITION PLAN

Once you complete your Reset nutrition plan you can now take control over what you eat. You should already have dropped some unwanted fat and should be feeling lighter. Follow the laws below to keep shredding fat and to achieving your health goals.

The Shred Fat Laws

1. Only choose foods that are on the lists as much as possible.
2. No processed foods or drinks.
3. No breads or refined flour.
4. Eat a protein at every meal.
5. Green vegetables should dominate the plate.
6. Re-feed after your workout.
7. Use herbs and spices freely to add flavour to your meals.
8. Eating breakfast in the morning is recommended.
9. Eat every 2 to 3 hours.
10. Prepare meals in advance if you have a busy lifestyle.
11. Drink at least 2 litres of water a day.
12. Take your Aloe Vera, fish oil and multi-vitamin and mineral every day.
13. Coffee and tea is limited to 2 cups a day, limit milk and no sugar. Use stevia as a sugar alternative.

Basically if a food has more than one ingredient then don't eat it!

Eating smaller meals frequently will increase your metabolism, making you a fat shredding machine. Choose the foods you like the most and that will be your shopping list. If it's not on the list, it is not in your basket. That goes for only food items by the way, don't use it as an excuse not to buy soap or deodorant!

We all fall off the wagon from time to time, but just refocus on your goal and get back up. Reward yourself after the 6 weeks with your close friends and enjoy an unhealthy meal. Life is for living.

This really isn't a 6-week program, it's a lifestyle program. Continue eating this way and you will be healthy. Anytime you stray from the program you can always come back and do the seven day Reset to get you back in the zone.

It's all in your mind-set to make good health decisions. Is instant gratification of chomping on McDonalds more important than the goal you put on paper? Only you can decide.

Choose only the foods provided on the lists below over the course of the next six weeks.

Eat as much as you like with every meal or snack:

- Broccoli
- Spinach

- Asparagus
- Kale
- Romaine Lettuce
- Collards
- Ginger
- Peas
- Ginger
- Garlic
- Bok Choi
- Cabbage
- Artichoke
- Celery
- Sprouts
- Chives
- Rocket
- Cucumber
- Peppers
- Green Beans
- Onions
- Eggplant
- Tomatoes
- Turnip
- Artichoke
- Carrots
- Zucchini

Eat one of the following proteins with every meal:

- Chicken
- Turkey
- Pork
- Lean Red Meat
- Wild Game
- Halibut
- Salmon
- Bacon
- Protein Shake
- Herring
- Cod

- Eggs
- Shrimp
- Anchovies
- Sardines

Eat one of the following carbohydrates with your post workout meal:

- Sweet Potato
- Oatmeal/ Oat Bran
- Hulled Barley
- Quinoa
- Brown Rice
- White Rice

Salad Dressings:

- Olive Oil
- Balsamic Vinegar
- Lemon Juice
- Coconut Oil
- Almond Oil
- Walnut Oil

Choose three of the following foods/drinks to consume once daily with your meals or snacks:

- Apple
- Banana
- Avocado
- Plain Yogurt
- Greek Yogurt
- Glass of Milk
- Handful of Unsalted Nuts/ Seeds
- Grapes
- Pineapple Slices
- Watermelon Slice

- Plum
- Orange
- Peach
- Blueberries/ Raspberries/ Blackberries
- 2 Squares Dark Chocolate
- Tbsp. Natural Almond Butter
- Tbsp. Natural Peanut Butter

Drink freely each day:

- Water
- Macha Tea
- Hibiscus Tea
- Nettle Tea
- Chamomile Tea
- Green Tea
- Peppermint Tea
- Ginger Tea

Supplements to take each day:

- Aloe Vera
- Fish Oil
- Multi Vitamin and Mineral
- Protein Shake (optional)

Cook with:

- Coconut Oil
- Grass-Fed Butter

SAMPLE DAY

Meal one
100ml Aloe Vera and a glass of water.
10 minutes later eat:
2 Egg omelette made with onion, garlic and red peppers.
2 fish oils capsules and a multivitamin and mineral

Snack one
Greek yogurt with 8 almonds and a green tea.

Meal two
Avocado salad with grilled chicken.
A Large glass of water.

Snack two
A freshly made Juice- Carrot, cucumber, ginger and apple.

Meal Three
Baked Salmon with Steamed Asparagus. If you worked out in the evening, you can add a baked sweet potato.
A glass of water and a camomile tea.

Summary

- The goal of this book is to shred fat and build muscle.
- Don't calorie restrict long term.
- Exercise is not essential in the seven-day Reset Phase, but that is not an excuse not to be active. Move, and move often.
- Get your life in balance (sleep, work, circle, nutrition, mindset), I can't stress enough how important these things are. I understand it is not easy for some but, achieving a balance may have to be a goal some of you have to work at daily.
- Increase your metabolism by building more muscle, eating smaller meals often, and by increasing your physical activity level.
- Follow the seven-day reset plan religiously.
- Eat only natural non-processed foods.
- Take Aloe Vera, fish oil and a multivitamin and mineral complex every single day.
- You can take a protein shake after workouts or if you skip a meal.
- Limit coffee to two cups a day
- Seven-day Reset phase includes two meals and three snacks.
- On the five-week Shred Phase, you can eat some extra complex carbohydrates after your workouts.
- Eat green vegetables at every meal.
- Cook with grass-fed butter and coconut oil only.
- Choose only foods from the lists provided.
- Go food shopping on a full stomach.
- Read the Labels.

TRAINING

TRAINING

On the Shred Fat Program, you will train four times a week, these include:

- Two strength training circuits
- Two Interval training workouts

Your weekly schedule will be as follows:

Day 1   Circuit A

Day 2   Interval

Day 3   Off

Day 4   Circuit B

Day 5   Interval

Day 6   Off

Day 7   Off

Choose which day of the week is your day one. This program has to work around your current lifestyle. For most, day one will be on Monday which gifts you the weekend to enjoy a nice active rest day with your family and friends. Having the weekend off is not an excuse to be hungover on Sunday morning with a breakfast roll watching the Coronation Street omnibus on BBC!

START A TRAINING DIARY

Buy a notebook or use your phone, but you have to record every training session. Keeping track of your training will show you where you are improving each week, and what exercises you need to work on. I find it is a great motivator when you flick back the pages to see how far you have come.

I'm very forgetful, I can't rely on my memory to know what weight I lifted or how many intervals I sprinted on my previous workout. A training dairy keeps me on track to make sure I'm always progressing. I'm engaged fully in my workouts when I'm at the gym. Before I start an exercise I already know what weight I need to lift and how many repetitions I need to do to better myself.

Write down as much information into the diary as possible. For example, if you have a great day in the gym and you smash all your previous records, then write down what led to that day.

- How where you feeling?
- What did you eat?
- How did you sleep the night before?
- Did you train earlier than usual?

This also works for your bad days. The aim is to find out what leads you to make the best progress in the gym and then follow that path to success.

At the start of your training dairy write down your short term goal, long term goal, waist measurement and weight. Each week update this information without fail.

A PROGRAM FOR EVERYBODY

It is impossible to design one program that suits everybody, because you will all have your own strengths, weaknesses and limitations. I have only prescribed exercises that most people should to some degree be able to perform. Proper technique is vital! Only progress to harder variations once you master the basics in this book. The basics are your bread and butter.

Nutrition is the most important aspect for shredding fat. Nutrition is the king and exercise is the queen. In Saudi, the kings have many queens and so do you. My training program is just one queen in a room of many queens. After six weeks, please join a kettlebell class, a TRX class, a spinning class or a pole dancing class. Just get moving and get active for variety is the spice of life. You have many queens waiting in their chambers, so visit each queen from time to time and drop the queens you don't like. If you love just one queen, great. But in the world of exercise, it's ok to be a polygamist.

PAIN

Pain is a sign that something is wrong. A lot of people choose to ignore pain and take a few painkillers and go about their day. You would be surprised with how many empty packets of pain pills I see in locker room bins. This can also lead to a physical dependence. Please go to a doctor to find the source of the pain, don't just cover up the symptoms by popping pills. Exercising through pain may exacerbate the issue and may make exercising harder in the future. You go to the mechanic when the engine light comes on, so go to the doctor when you have pain.

ALWAYS WARM-UP

You must warm-up before every workout. This is not just a ten-minute walk on the treadmill playing solitaire. So on that note leave your phone in your gym bag and get shit done. You can post gym selfies to Instagram after your workout.

Each warm-up will take approximately fifteen minutes to complete. The Shred Fat warm-up will increase mobility of your joints, improve your posture, increase flexibility and will reduce your risk of injury significantly.

The warm up consists of eight soft tissue manipulation exercises and eight mobility and stability drills. The soft tissue work will be the same every workout session while you alternate the mobility and stability drills each workout.

SOFT TISSUE WORK

There is a soft connective tissue just below our skin called superficial fascia. These tissues connect and wrap bones, muscles, blood vessels and nerves in the body. This fascia becomes stuck to underlying muscles. When this fascia sticks to a muscle it is called an adhesion or a knot. These adhesions limit range of motion, and if you exercise with them you are increasing your chances of injury tenfold.

You need a solid foundation of pliable connective tissue. Doing soft tissue exercises before training helps to free up this connective tissue giving you better range of motion, relieving muscle soreness, increasing flexibility and will improve overall connective tissue health.

Foam rollers, tennis balls and steel bars are the best pieces of equipment to work your soft tissue. You are essentially giving your body a massage before exercising.

Don't skip your eight soft tissue exercises at the start of each workout. I recommend to do them every day if you have flexibility or movement issues. I have chosen these eight because they hit many different areas of the body and you will get the best bang for your buck.

Tips for soft tissue work

- Use your body weight as much as possible, put as much pressure into the roller/ball/bar as possible.
- Don't hold your breath, just breath normally and relax your muscles into the roller/ball/bar.

- Explore around the muscle area to pin point these adhesions, once found keep the pressure on this painful area until the pain diminishes about 50% (exercise shouldn't hurt, but these adhesions can be painful at first, so start of easy).
- Do approximately 45 seconds for each soft tissue exercise.

The eight soft tissue exercises are:

1. Quad Roll
2. Hip-flexor Roll
3. Back Roll
4. Lat Smash
5. Glute Medius Roll
6. Adductor Roll
7. Hamstring Smash
8. Calf Smash

Proceed to exercise section to view the soft tissue exercises.

MOBILITY AND STABILITY DRILLS

The second part of your warm up is doing eight mobility and stability drills. I have created two different sets of these drills which will improve your posture significantly. You will be moving better and feeling better in no time.

Soft tissue work and the mobility and stability drills before every workout will prepare your body for the circuits and interval training. Adhesions will go away and connective tissue and joint health will dramatically improve.

The drills will work your joints through their full range of motion. Get into the habit of doing these drills daily. If you sit at your desk all day in work, then its beneficial to stand up every 30 minutes and do some of these drills. The more you foam roll and do these drills, the better you will move. That I promise you.

Mobility and stability drills set 1:

1. Arm Swing Matrix
2. Lateral Leg Swings
3. Hamstring Mobilizer
4. Bird Dog
5. Wall Slides

6. Cat Stretch
7. Frog Stretch
8. Bridges

Mobility and stability drills set 2:

1. Arm Swing Matrix
2. Frontal Leg Swings
3. Wall Stretch
4. Thoracic Rotations
5. Pigeon Pose
6. Downward Facing Dog
7. Glute Stretch
8. Cobra

CIRCUIT TRAIN

I love circuit training because you train upper and lower body in every training session. You will train all the large muscle groups; and in turn the small muscles, like the biceps will also grow. Doing bicep curls as stand-alone exercises are good for your ego, but they don't do much for your metabolic rate or muscle mass.

The leg muscles are the biggest muscles in the body, only training them once a week makes no sense. By training them in every circuit, you will increase your testosterone levels and maximize muscle gains in all parts of your body.

Alternate between the two circuits each week. The circuits I created have safety in mind, so I haven't included exercises like back squats or full deadlifts because I'm not there to test your movement limitations or assess your movement efficiency. I have included simple exercises that train the body as a whole.

Your two circuits will be as follows:

Circuit A

1. Split Squat
2. Hamstring Curl
3. Lat Pulldown
4. Push Ups
5. Landmines

6. Leg Raise
7. Burpees

Circuit B

1. Dumbbell Deadlift
2. Goblet Squat
3. Chest Press
4. Cable Rows
5. Lean and Press
6. Plank
7. Mountain Climbers

LIFT BIG

This goes for both men and women. The more muscle mass you have the faster your Resting Metabolic Rate increases, helping you burn more calories daily. Gaining or maintaining as much muscle mass as possible is a must in order to shred fat.

To get those muscles you have to lift heavy weights. Don't worry about looking like Arnold, you won't. Lifting heavy twice a week with a repetition range between 8 to 10 reps has worked wonders with my clients. If you can manage more than 10 reps on any exercise, then it is time to increase the weight. You will record all this information in your training diary.

Only count proper repetitions, I'm very strict on form in my gym. If you don't think you can get another quality rep, then don't even try. Leave it for the next time. Safety is paramount.

THE BURN OUT

At the end of each circuit you will do two sets of a burn out exercise. The two burn out exercises on this program are:

• Burpees
• Mountain Climbers

Burn outs are a great way to increase your metabolic rate. They are perfect to do at the very end so you can put as much effort into the exercise as possible knowing you can relax once they are finished. The goal is to get as many reps as possible in 60 seconds. You may only get a few but as the weeks go on keep recording the number you get in your diary and always try to better yourself each week.

TEMPO

The speed at which you lower and lift a weight affects the results you will get. There are two types of muscle contraction you need to understand, concentric and eccentric contractions.

Eccentric contractions are the lengthening of a muscle while producing force. For example, during a chest press, you will lower the weight slowly from the top position until the bar nearly touches your chest. You are essentially slowing down the weight instead of allowing the weight to just fall.

Concentric is simply the shortening of a muscle against a resistive force. For example, during the chest press when you have eccentrically lowered the weight to your chest, the concentric contraction is when you push the bar up to the starting position, shortening your pectoral muscles.

The tempo for your lifts are 3-1-3. Three seconds concentric/eccentric and a one second pause in between the two contractions. If you are doing 8 repetitions, that's 56 seconds of time under tension. This will increase your metabolic rate by building muscle mass and increasing physical activity level, all leading to fat burning.

PROGRESSIONS

I want you to start off light and practice the technique of each exercise. Use your bodyweight at the beginning if the exercise permits, then start adding external resistance. You must recognize when to make an exercise harder and progress to either a heavier weight or a different variation of the exercise.

All exercises have progressions to make an exercise more challenging. For example, the plank (included in exercise list). The plank is a great exercise when done properly but I see many trainers having their clients holding the plank for far too long. Thirty to forty seconds is enough time to hold a plank. If forty seconds is too easy for you, it is not more time you need, it's a more challenging way of doing the exercise. Placing your elbows on a fit ball with your feet on the floor is a common progression. The time remains the same but you have just increased the difficulty of the exercise.

Again, master good form first before progressing.

ACTIVE REST BETWEEN SETS

When strength training heavy you have to rest for 60 seconds between sets to give your muscles and nervous system time to recover. Use these 60 seconds wisely, the majority of gym users waste this time watching the TV, looking at their phones and scratching their asses.

My clients stretch, foam roll or do some mobility drills in between sets. It keeps them focused on the task at hand and they will make better improvements in the long run if they constantly work on themselves. If you're not drinking water, then choose an exercise from our warm up and get the most out of your rest period. Your body will thank you in the long run.

INTERVALS

You are required to do two interval training sessions a week. Intervals are amazing at burning calories and the best thing of all is that they don't require a large amount of your time. Choose a cardio exercise you like so it will be easier to stick to the program.

Choose one of the following exercises:

- Sprinting (treadmill/outside)
- Rower
- Stationary Bike
- Airdyne Bike
- Skipping
- Swim Sprints

Everybody is different so you need to set your speed, duration and rest based on your level. Start off with a work/rest ratio of 1:2 in the first two weeks.

- Beginners should start with 30 seconds of work with 60 seconds rest.
- Intermediate should start with 45 seconds of work with 90 seconds rest.
- Advanced should start with 60 seconds of work with 120 seconds of rest.

Work = As hard and as fast as you can possibly go.

Rest = Do absolutely nothing, don't pedal slow or walk. Just focus on breathing and recovering.

Every two weeks keep the work the same while decreasing the rest. By the last two weeks we are aiming for 1:1 work/rest ratio. If you can manage a 1:1 work/rest ratio from week one then by all means go for it, make this program your own.

The Workout:

1. Warm up: soft tissue, mobility and stability exercises and add a 5 minute cardio exercise at a moderate pace.
2. Main Phase: 6-8 rounds of Intervals.
3. Cool down: 3-5 minute cardio exercise at a slow pace.

For Beginners, the 6 weeks will look like this:

Weeks 1-2:
30 seconds high intensity work, 60 seconds rest. Repeat for 6-8 rounds.

Weeks 3-4:
30 seconds high intensity work, 45 seconds rest. Repeat for 6-8 rounds.

Weeks 5-6:
30 seconds high intensity work, 30 seconds rest. Repeat for 6-8 rounds.

Log your results in your training diary. Write down what level you used on a machine, how many reps per minute you pedaled, how you felt, heart rate etc. If it's in the training diary you will know what adjustments to make on the next session.

WORKOUT 1 AND 3

Warm Up:

1. Quad Roll – 45 seconds
2. Hip-Flexor Roll- 45 seconds each side
3. Back Roll- 45 seconds
4. Lat Smash- 45 seconds each side
5. Glute Medius Roll- 45 seconds each side
6. Adductor Roll- 45 seconds each side
7. Hamstring Smash- 45 seconds each side
8. Calf Smash- 45 seconds each side

1. Arm Swing Matrix- 10 reps of each
2. Lateral Leg Swings- 10 reps each side
3. Hamstring Mobilizer- 10 reps each side
4. Bird Dog- 10 reps each side
5. Wall Slides- 10 reps
6. Cat Stretch- 10 reps
7. Frog Stretch- 10 reps
8. Bridges- 10 reps

Then continue to do Circuit A or circuit B.

Circuit A

Exercise	Sets	Reps	Tempo	Rest in between sets
Split Squat	3	8 to 10	3-1-3	60 seconds
Hamstring Curl	3	8 to 10	3-1-3	60 seconds
Lat pulldown	3	8 to 10	3-1-3	60 seconds
Push ups	2	MAX	1-0-1	60 seconds
Landmines	2	8 to 10	2-1-1	30 seconds
Leg raise	2	8 to 10	1-0-1	30 seconds
Burpees	2	MAX	FAST	60 seconds

Circuit B

Exercise	Sets	Reps	Tempo	Rest in between sets
Dumbbell Deadlift	3	8 to 10	3-0-3	60 seconds
Goblet Squat	3	8 to 10	3-1-3	60 seconds
Bench Press	2	8 to 10	3-1-3	60 seconds
Cable Rows	3	8 to 10	3-1-3	60 seconds
Lean and Press	3	8 to 10	3-1-3	60 seconds
Plank	2	MAX	HOLD	30 seconds
Mountain Climbers	2	MAX	FAST	60 seconds

Record all weights and reps in your training diary

WORKOUT 2 AND 4

Warm Up:

Quad Roll – 45 seconds

1. Hip-Flexor Roll- 45 seconds each side
2. Back Roll- 45 seconds
3. Lat Smash- 45 seconds each side
4. Glute Medius Roll- 45 seconds each side
5. Adductor Roll- 45 seconds each side
6. Hamstring Smash- 45 seconds each side
7. Calf Smash- 45 seconds each side

1. Arm Swing Matrix- 10 reps of each
2. Frontal Leg Swings- 10 reps each side
3. Wall Stretch- 45 seconds stretch on each side
4. Thoracic Rotations- 10 reps each side
5. Pigeon Pose- 45 seconds stretch on each side
6. Downward Facing Dog- 30 seconds stretch
7. Glute Stretch- 30-45 seconds stretch on each side
8. Cobra- 30 second stretch on each side

5 minute slow pace on the cardio machine you choose. Then do 6-8 rounds of Intervals on cardio machine of your choice.

Sample:

Weeks 1-2:
30 seconds high intensity work, 60 seconds rest. Repeat for 6-8 rounds.

Weeks 3-4:
30 seconds high intensity work, 45 seconds rest. Repeat for 6-8 rounds.

Weeks 5-6:
30 seconds high intensity work, 30 seconds rest. Repeat for 6-8 rounds.
Cool down: 3-5 minute cardio exercise at a slow pace.

Summary

- You will Train 4 times a week, 2 circuit training sessions and 2 interval training sessions.
- Start a training Diary.
- Pain means STOP!! Go see a doctor.
- Always warm-up (Soft tissue/ Mobility and Stability drills)
- Technique is paramount, before adding weight make sure you can execute the technique properly and safely. Ask a trainer in the gym if you need assistance.
- Lift heavy weights.
- Repetition range between 8 to 10.
- Do 2 sets of a burn out exercise at the end of every circuit.
- Follow the tempo, work the eccentric contraction just as much as the concentric.
- Use exercise progressions.
- Make the most of your rest between sets, use some mobility drills from the warmup while you wait for your next set.
- Ease into interval training if it is new to you and choose an exercise you enjoy.
- Start off with a 1:2 work/rest ratio for interval training working up to 1:1.

EXERCISE

(1) Quad Roll

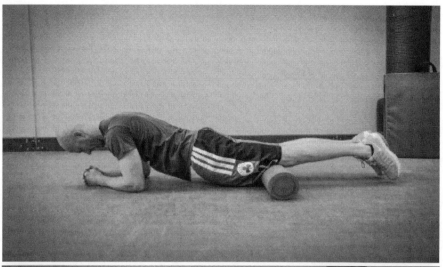

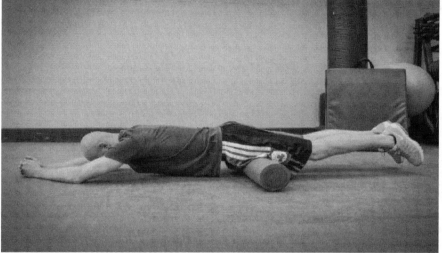

A basic foam rolling exercise to free up the connective tissue around the quadriceps. If you have tight connective tissue, foam rolling will be slightly painful. Over time the pain will subside.

- Position the foam roller just above your knee cap, with your elbows under your shoulders.
- Use your elbows to roll slowly up and down the length of the quadriceps, searching for tight painful connective tissue.
- Keep your core engaged.
- Relax your breathing.

(2) Hip-Flexor Roll

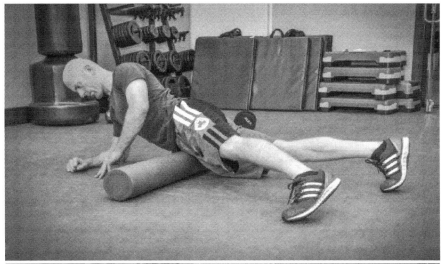

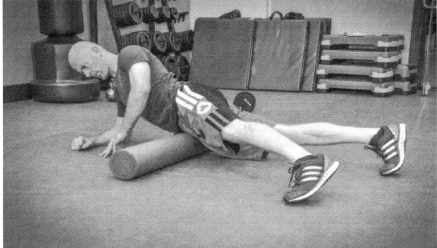

Tight hips are very common, because of all the sitting we do daily. This exercise will hit your hip-flexor to free up this connective tissue.

- With your right leg fully extended, position the foam roller on your right psoas major (muscle just below your waistline).
- Turn your torso away from the roller, and put as much weight as possible onto the muscle.
- Slowly roll up and down, and side to side searching for tight spots in the area.
- Stay relaxed and breath normally.
- Repeat both sides.

(3) Back Roll

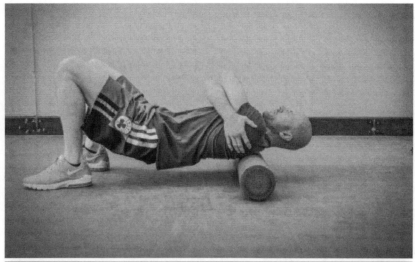

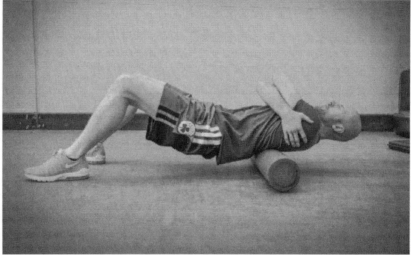

Great for hitting tight connective tissue on the upper and middle back.

- Lying on the floor, position the foam roller on the top of your shoulder blades.
- With your feet close to your hips, lift your hips off the floor.
- Hug your body with your arms.
- Push your feet into the floor to foam roll up and down your spine.
- Keep the pressure on any tight areas, avoid the lumbar spine if you are a beginner.
- You can also lean side to side slowly on any tight, painful areas.
- Relaxed breathing.

(4) Lat Smash

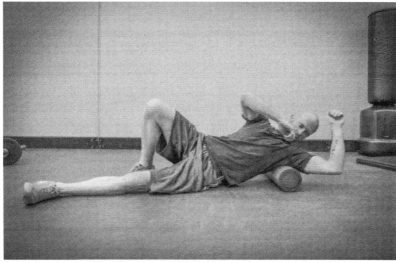

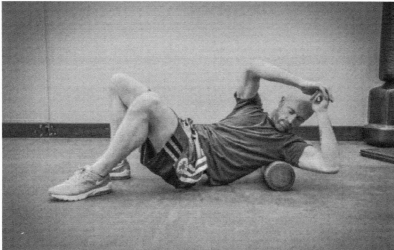

Knots are very common in the latissimus dorsi region. This can lead to shoulder and back pain. Freeing up these areas are crucial to reduce your risk of injuries.

- Position the foam roller at the back of your armpit.
- Put as much weight as possible on the muscle with your left leg straight.
- If you don't feel much, bend your left knee and lift your hip off the floor, this will add more pressure on the area.
- Roll up and down and side to side to search for tight spots.
- Repeat both sides.

(5) Glute Medius Roll

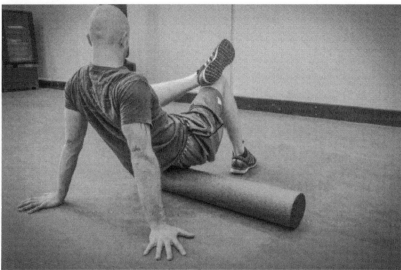

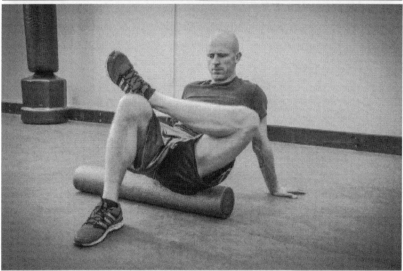

The glute medius is also very prone to knots. They can be hard to locate a first, but you will know all about it when you find it, as they are painful. Freeing up this area will help you move better, period.

- Sit on a foam roller with one leg crossed over the other.
- If your left leg is crossed, lean slightly to the left.
- Sink into the roller.
- Search for knots and tight areas by slowly rolling up and down and side to side.
- Repeat the opposite side.

(6) Adductor roll

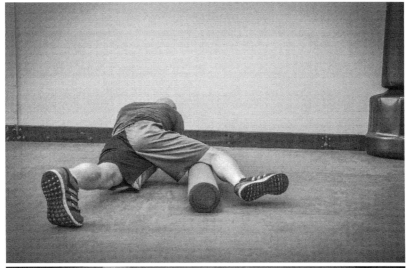

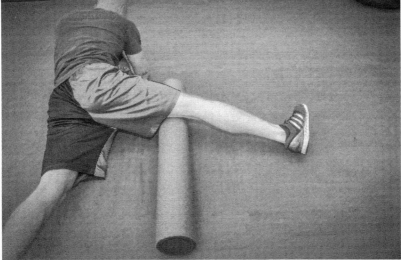

Tight adductors (inner thigh muscles) lead to hip mobility issues and movement dysfunctions. This exercise will increase your joint range of motion and improve movement quality.

- Place the inside of your right knee on a foam roller, left leg extended.
- Roll slowly up towards the middle of your thigh, putting as much weight as possible on the muscles of the inside leg.
- You can also flex and extend your right knee (shown in picture two).
- Search around the area for tight connective tissue. The more weight you put on the roller, the better.
- Repeat both sides.

(7) Hamstring Smash

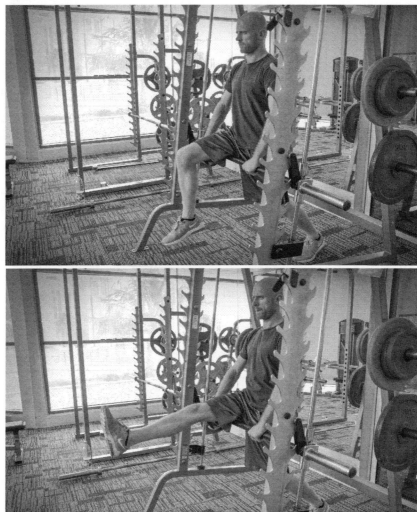

Hands down the best soft tissue exercise for your hamstrings. If you can't touch your toes, then this is an exercise for you.

- Position the meat of your upper hamstring onto a bar, relax into the bar putting as much weight as is bare-able.
- Flex and extend your knee, while keeping the pressure on the hamstring.
- Find tight spots by searching around the length of the hamstring by positioning the bar on different areas.
- Try also internally and externally rotating your leg to hit the hamstrings from different angles.
- No pain faces and relaxed breathing.

(8) Calf Smash

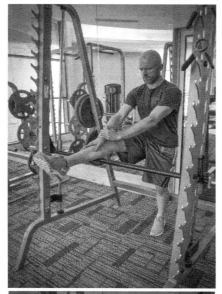

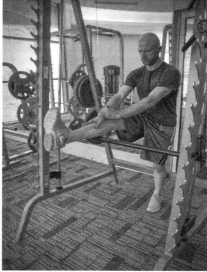

If you run or have overly tight calf muscles, then this Calf Smash will alleviate symptoms and restore tissue health.

- Place the bar on the meaty part of your calf muscle, and let the muscle sink into the bar.
- Flex and extend your foot to help free up the connective tissue.
- Turn your leg side to side to help hit the area from different angles.
- Search around the muscle to find tight spots.
- Push your hands into your calf to add extra pressure if required.
- As always, relaxed breathing.

(9) Arm Swing Matrix

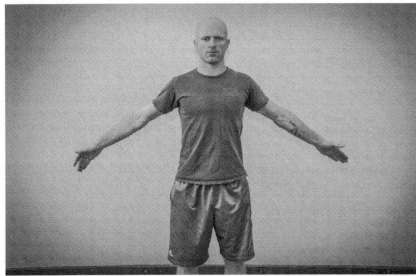

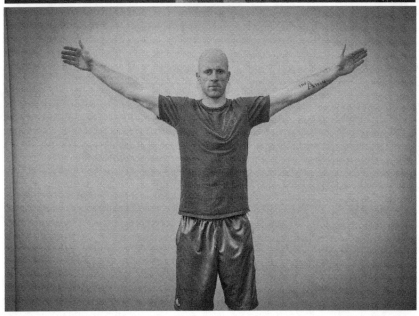

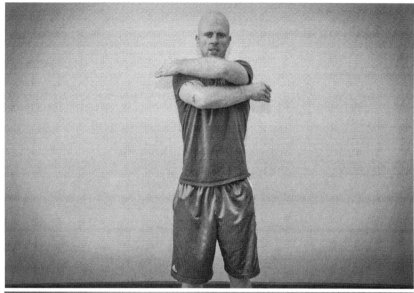

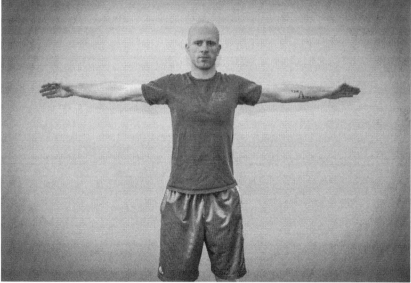

Free up the shoulder joint before each workout is a must, that's why the arm matrix is included in both sets of warmups.

- 10 big arm swing circles forward.
- 10 big arm swings backwards.
- 10 big arm swings side to side.
- Keep your back straight and head up.
- Swing to your full range of motion with speed.

(10) Lateral Leg Swings

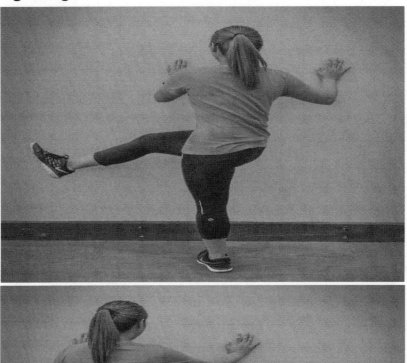

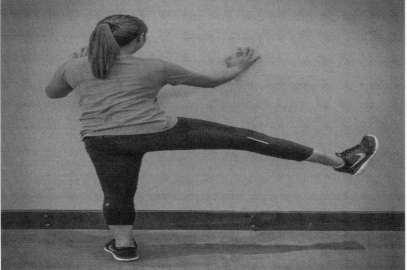

Good dynamic exercise to increase your range of motion in the hips and to improve circulation to the muscles.

- Toes of left foot facing the wall, back straight.
- Swing your right foot to the side, away from your left foot.
- Point right toes towards the ceiling.
- Then swing your right foot across your body, also pointing your toes towards the ceiling.
- Swing to your full range of motion with some speed.
- Repeat both sides.

(11) Hamstring Mobilizer

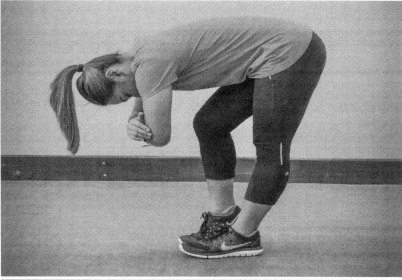

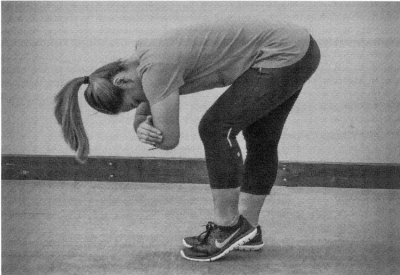

You will feel this in the tightest area of your posterior chain. For most it is in the hamstring but you may feel it on the back of your calves.

- With your left leg bent and right leg straight, fold forward from the hips until you feel a stretch on the back of your right leg.
- Slowly alternate by straightening the left leg while bending the right leg.
- Keep your head in line with your spine
- The focus should be on the hamstrings, so no unnecessary spinal flexion.

(12) Bird Dog

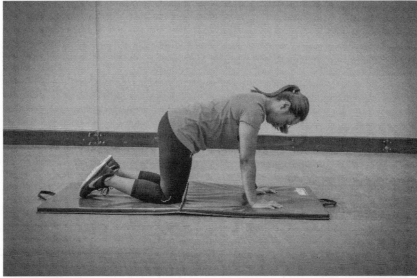

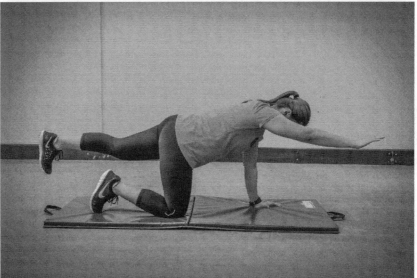

Full body stability drill which will work your balance, lower back and core.

- Start from the table position, which is hands directly under shoulders, and knees under hips.
- Slowly extend your left leg behind you while reaching your right arm forward.
- Don't lift your left leg higher than hip level or you will put your lumbar spine out of a good position.
- Keep head in line with the spine at all times.
- Return to table position and repeat with opposite arm and leg.

(13) Wall Slides

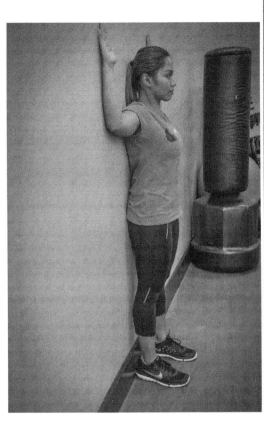 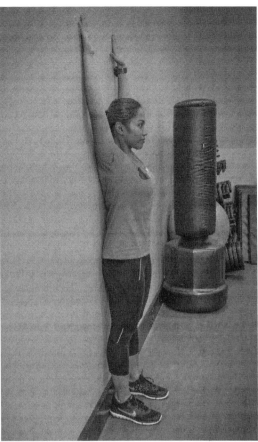

This exercise is my go to for thoracic spine mobility. Freeing up the T-spine can alleviate back pain, and will help improve efficiency in overhead movements.

- Stand with your back against a wall with a neutral spine.
- Place your hands and elbows on the wall.
- Slowly slide your hands up the wall, trying to keep your elbows and hands in contact with the wall without moving your spine.
- The gap between your lower back and the wall should remain the same throughout the movement.
- Work within your range of motion.

(14) Cat Stretch

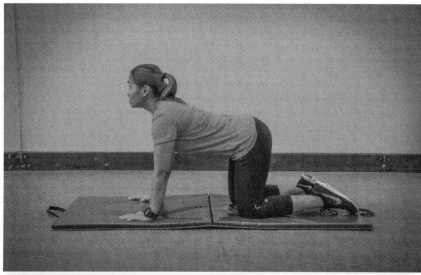

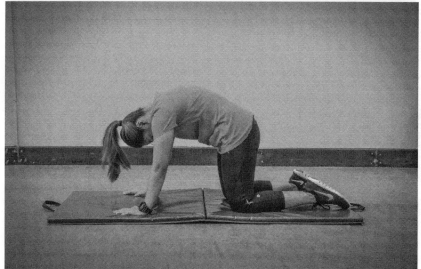

Great exercise in mobilizing the spine. This should be done every day, even more so if you are stuck in an office chair for eight hours of the day.

- From a table position, breath in and look up while pushing your belly button to the floor extending your spine.
- Then breath out slowly and flex your spine to the ceiling while looking at your knees.
- Repeat this movement in sync with your breathing.
- Don't force this exercise, just flow through your range of motion. Over time you will see and feel improvements.

(15) Frog Stretch

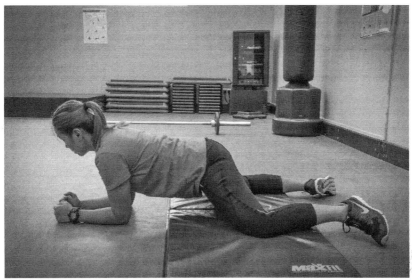

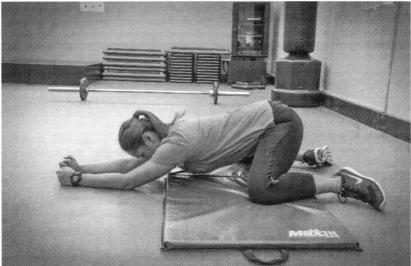

The number one inside groin stretch. This stretch will open up your hips and will improve flexibility.

- On a mat, spread your knees as wide as possible with your hips in front of your knees.
- Place your elbows under your shoulders and take a deep breath in.
- Push your elbows into the floor and breath out slowly while moving your hips back behind your knees.
- Spread your knees wider if you don't feel a stretch when your hips are behind your knees.
- Repeat for the desired repetitions.

(16) Bridges

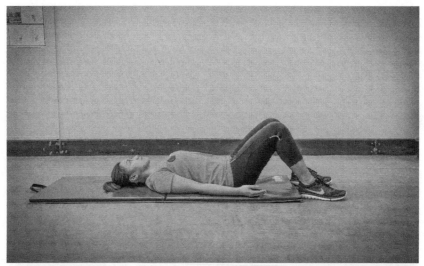

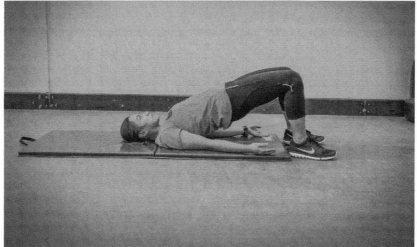

Bridges are a great glute activation exercise. Waking up your glutes before your workout will reduce your chance of injury, and will ensure that they fire when called upon.

- Lie on a mat, feet hip distance apart and feet close to your glutes.
- Driving through your heels, lift your hips off the mat by contracting your glutes as hard as you can.
- Slowly lower to the starting position.

Note: The main focus should not be lifting your hips, but on pushing your heels into the floor. Focus on squeezing your glutes as hard as you can at the top of the movement. This will eliminate the firing of the lower back muscles.

(17) Frontal Leg Swings

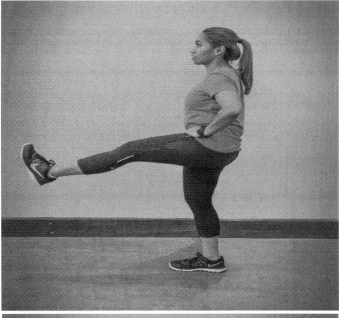

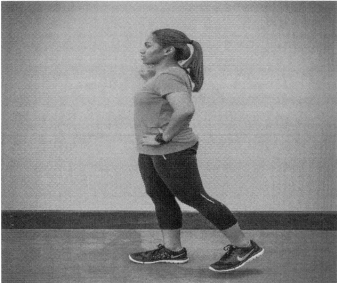

Great dynamic movement to open up the hips.

- Place your right hand on the wall for support.
- With a straight spine, swing your left leg as high as you can in front of you with speed.
- On the down swing, only go just behind your left leg as to not impact the lumbar spine.
- Do both sides.

(18) Wall Stretch

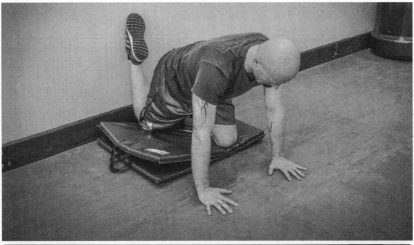

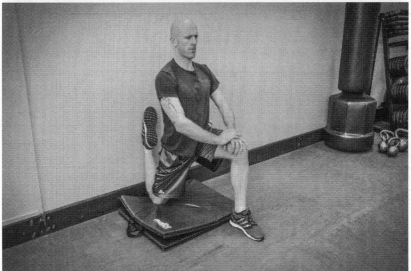

The ultimate hip flexor/quadriceps stretch. It will be painful if done right, but it is extremely effective.

- To get into this position, place your two knees on a mat and your hands on the floor.
- Place the top of your right foot on the wall and then step forward with your left leg.
- Place your hands on your right thigh and lean forward.
- Hold for desired time.
- Repeat the opposite side.

The closer your knee is to the wall, the more of a stretch you will get on your quadriceps and hip-flexors. Find the right distance for you.

(19) Thoracic Rotations

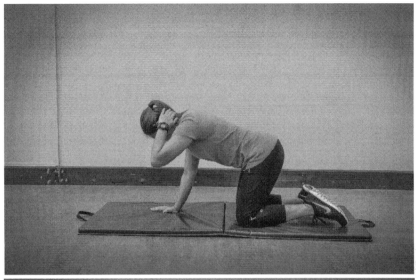

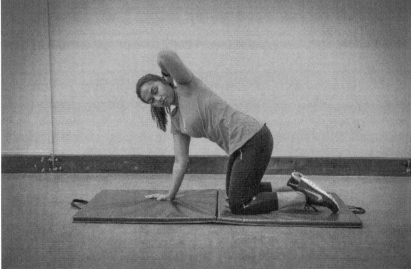

Improving the mobility of your T-spine will reduce your risk of lower back injuries. This drill immobilizes your hips, so the rotation must come from your T-spine.

- From a 3-point table position, look at the floor and have your left hand on your head.
- Rotate to your left, aiming to point your elbow towards the ceiling.
- Return to start position.
- Controlled, relaxed breathing throughout.
- Repeat the opposite side.

(20) Pigeon Pose

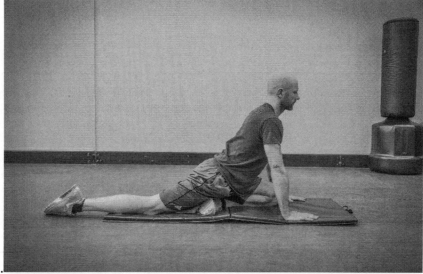

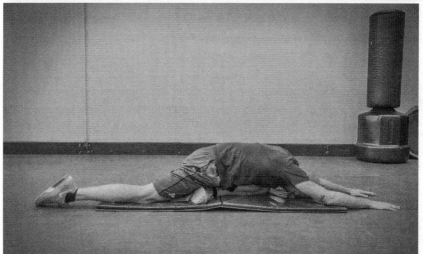

A beautiful hip opener stretch. It will stretch your hip flexors and hip rotator muscles.

- Start in a table position, hands under the shoulders and the knees under the hips.
- Place your left knee between your two hands, left foot under the right hip.
- Then, slide and stretch the right leg back.
- Hips stay square and the laces of your right foot facing the floor.
- To to go further into the stretch: walk your hands up the floor and lower your chest, and head to the mat.
- Relaxed breathing. Every time you breathe out sink deeper into the stretch.
- Repeat opposite side

(21) Downward Facing Dog

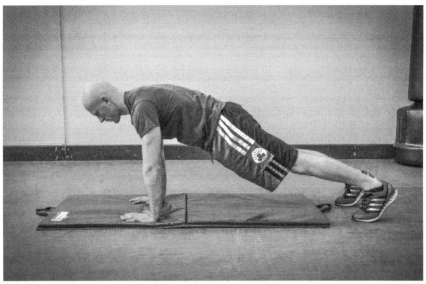

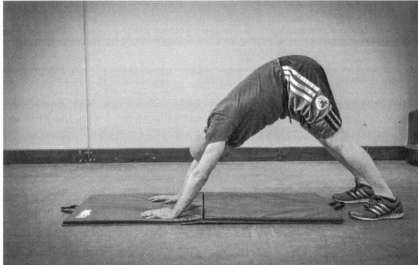

Free up tension in your hamstrings, calves, glutes, and back muscles all in one. It is no wonder that this exercise is in every yoga practice session.

- From the push up starting position, push your hands into the floor and lift your hips towards the ceiling.
- Look at your feet.
- Dig your heels into the floor.
- Beginners may bend their knees slightly.
- Hold for time and sink into the stretch while focusing on your breathing.

(22) Glute Stretch

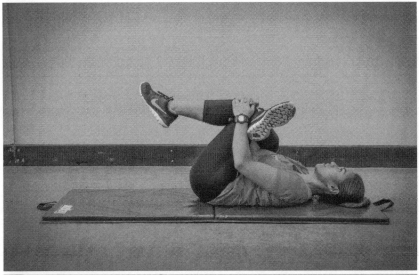

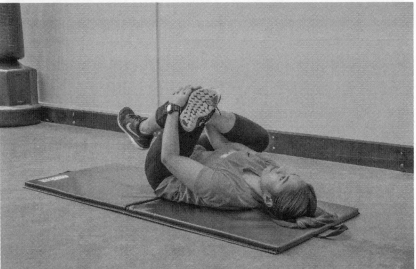

The classic glute stretch. This stretch increases flexibility of the hips. It's a perfect stretch after foam rolling your glute medius.

- Lie on a mat with knees bent.
- Place your right leg on your left knee.
- Lift your left knee towards your chest.
- Interlock your fingers and pull your left knee close to your chest.
- Relax your breathing and hold for time.
- Keep your head on the mat.
- Repeat the opposite side.

(23) Cobra

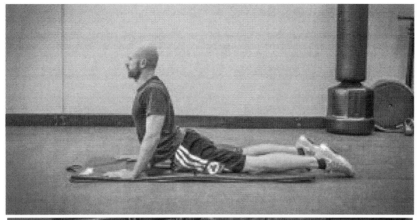

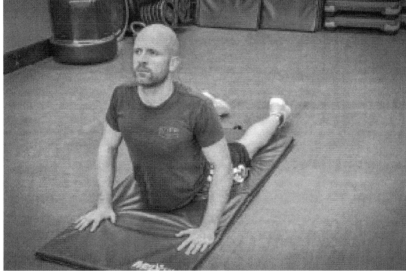

Backbends like the cobra pose are important for a healthy spine. It's a great stretch for the abdomen.

- Lie face down on the mat, with your hands under your shoulders.
- Engage your lower back muscles and lightly push your hands into the floor to lift your chest off the floor.
- Squeeze your glutes and push the hips into the floor for the duration of this pose.
- Roll your shoulders back to open your chest.
- Look straight ahead.
- Relaxed breathing.

If any pain/discomfort in the lower back during this pose, walk the hands further forward to relieve tension.

(24) Split Squat

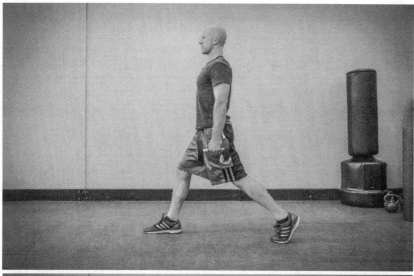

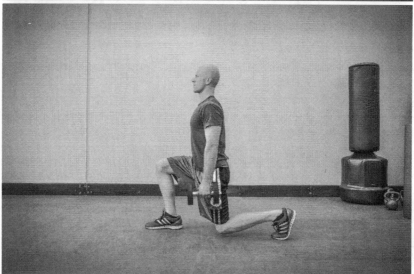

Not everybody has the movement quality to back squat. The split squat is a safe alternative; it is easy to keep your spine in alignment, which dramatically reduces your risk of injuries.

- Position your feet in a staggered stance.
- Hold a dumbbell in each hand, arms straight.
- Bend your front knee and lower your body down while keeping your back straight.
- Keep your front knee over your front heel. In the bottom position, the angle at the back of both knees should be approximately 90 degrees
- At the bottom, drive through your front foot to return to the start position.

(25) Hamstring Curl

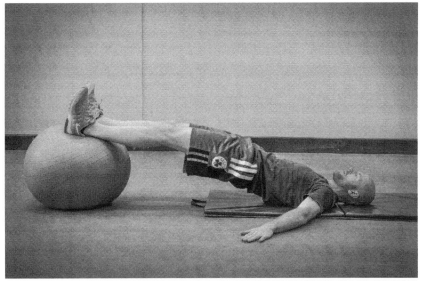

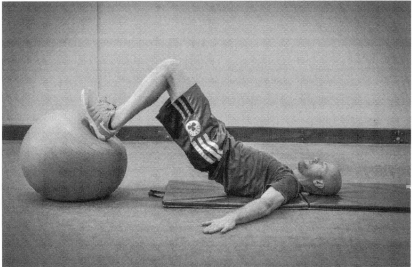

Incredible exercise to strengthen the hamstrings with the added benefit of working on your core stability.

- Lie on a mat and place your feet on a medium sized fit-ball.
- Drive your heels down into the fit-ball and lift your hips by contracting your glutes.
- Keep your abs tight, pull the ball towards your glutes while really focusing on squeezing your glutes and hamstrings.
- Push the ball away from your glutes to return to the start position.

(26) Lat Pulldown

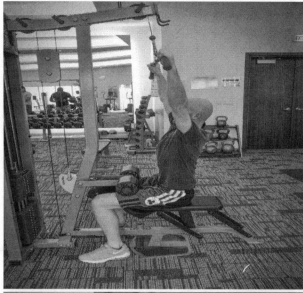

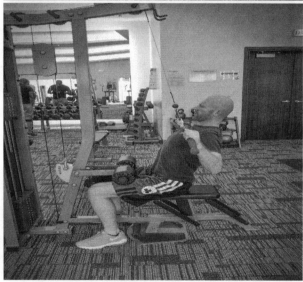

Pull ups are great, but not everybody can manage their own weight. So start off on a Lat pulldown machine. I don't use many machines with my clients, but this is one of the exceptions.

- Grab the bar a little wider than shoulder width and sit down with feet hip distance apart, back straight and core engaged.
- Lean back slightly while pulling the bar to your collar bone.
- Squeeze your shoulder blades together when the bar touches your chest.
- Return to the start position.

(27) Push Ups

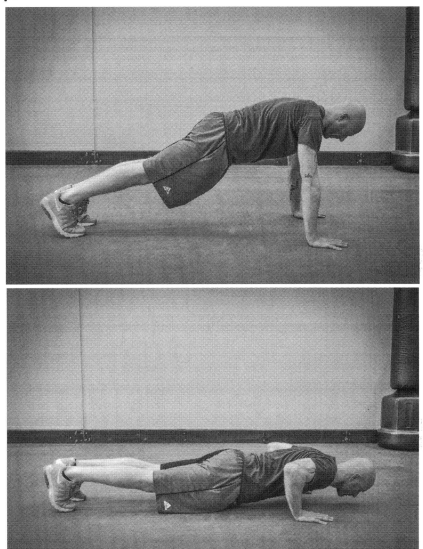

One of the best exercises on the planet. All of my clients do push-ups every week, and you will do the same. Not only are you working your chest, but you are working a lot of stabilizer muscles too.

- Start with your hands shoulder width apart, with abs and glutes engaged.
- Slowly lower your chest to the floor keeping your hips, shoulders and head in line.
- Push through your hands while breathing out, returning to the start position.

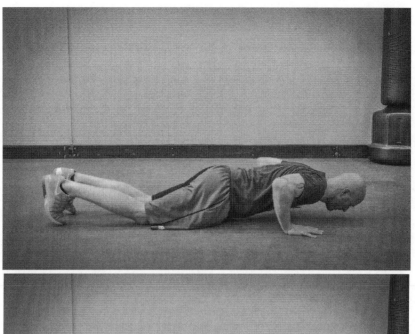

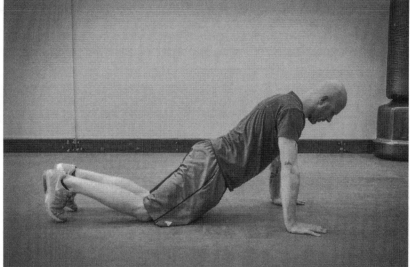

Doing full push-ups may be hard, so instead follow all 4 pictures.

- Start in a full push up and lower to the floor, working the eccentric contraction and handling your bodyweight.
- Then if you cannot do a push up from the bottom, place your knees on the floor and push your hands into the floor, keeping your abs and glutes always engaged.
- Then lift your knees so you are back to the starting position.

Working the eccentric contraction will lead to full pushups over time. Refrain from just knee on floor push-ups unless absolutely necessary.

(28) Landmines

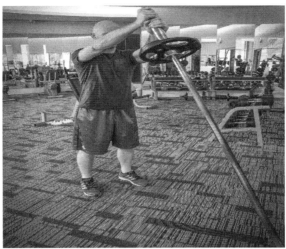

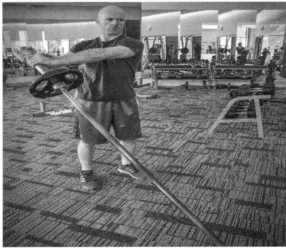

This is a tremendous anti-rotation exercise. I see many people doing this exercise with lots of upper body movement which is wrong. Your goal is to limit upper body movement by engaging your core to not rotate.

- Place an Olympic bar into a corner or landmine device.
- Raise the bar off the floor so the bar is a little higher than shoulder height, and your arms are extended.
- Bend your knees slightly and keep your spine upright.
- Using your arms, move the bar to the side without moving your upper body.
- Use your core to not rotate and to pull the bar back to the start position.
- Breath in when the bar goes to the side and out when you are back in the start position.
- Alternate between both sides for the desired amount of reps.

(29) Leg Raise

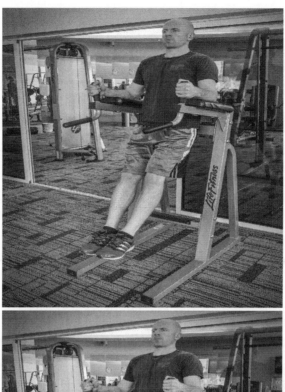

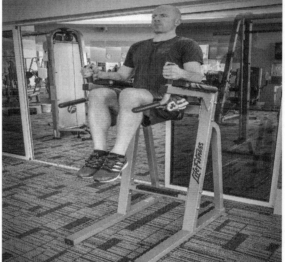

Great core strengthening exercise with no unnecessary spinal flexion.

- Place your elbows on a leg raise machine and position your back firmly on the pad.
- Hang vertical to the floor with your feet hanging, point your toes straight down.
- Lift your knees to be in line with your hips while breathing in.
- Then slowly lower to start position while breathing out.

If 10 reps become too easy, then progress to a straight leg variation.

(30) Burpees

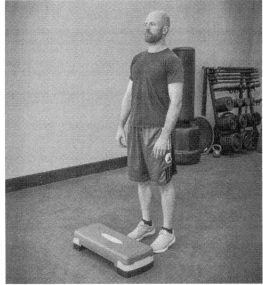

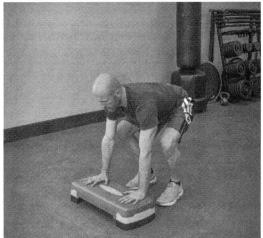

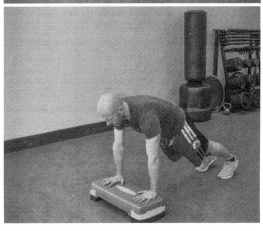

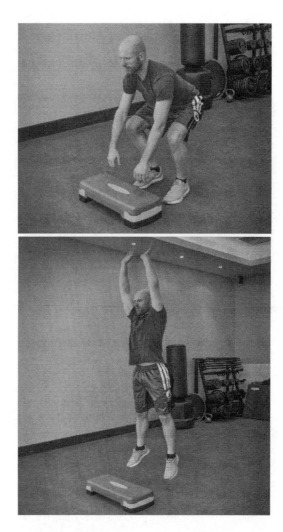

The most dreaded exercise in my gym. Burpees train your body as a whole. They will burn a lot of calories and increase your metabolic rate, so don't skip them at the end!

- Stand with your hips shoulder width apart and back straight, engage your core.
- Hinge forward at the hips, knees go out and place hands on the platform/floor.
- Jump your feet back into a starting push up position- abs and glutes engaged.
- Jump back to your hands, and take your hands off the platform at the same time, so you end up in a good bottom squat position with a straight spine.
- Jump explosively into the air from the squat position.
- Land in the starting stance and repeat for time.

Keep your back flat when you bend down. The platform can be any height you wish, focus on good form. Look at the pictures carefully and look at foot position, spine alignment, head position and arm position in each photo. The end goal is doing burpees with no platform.

(31) Dumbbell Deadlift

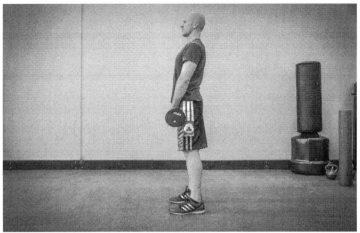

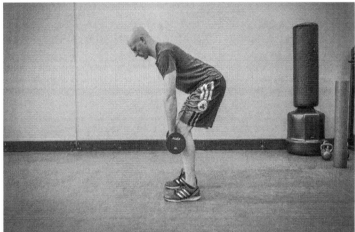

The Dumbbell Deadlift is beginner friendly. Pay close attention to the pictures. Master this one over the 6-weeks before progressing to harder variations.

- Stand with your back straight, hip distance apart and dumbbells in front of the hips.
- Abs engaged and squeeze the dumbbells tight.
- Hinge at the hips (like sitting back).
- Lower the dumbbells to just below your kneecap.
- Head stays in line with the spine and abs always engaged.
- Contract your glutes, push your heels into the floor and push your hips forward.
- Repeat for desired reps.

Always keep your core engaged and control the eccentric and concentric contraction. The movement comes from your hips and not from your knees. Imagine you are about to sit down and then change your mind. Limit any spinal flexion!

(32) Goblet Squat

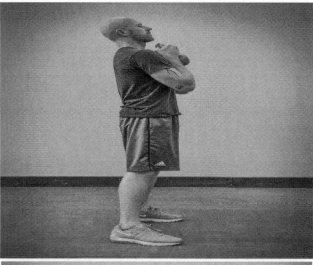

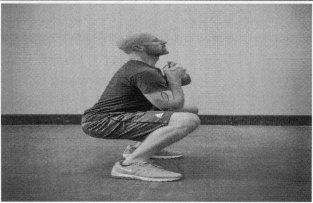

The goblet squat is a beautiful exercise. It will reinforce good movement mechanics, and it will help you squat better in the future. Master this basic movement pattern before moving onto normal squats. Don't go heavy, just work on the technique!

- Hold a kettlebell in your hands, elbows under hands, and place your feet shoulder width apart.
- Squat down while keeping your pelvis tucked in, go as low as you can without leaning forward.
- Heels must remain on the floor at all times.
- Hold for a second in the bottom position with elbows inside of your knees.
- Then drive through your feet while squeezing your glutes as much as possible returning to the start position.

Some of you may be able to lower all the way down and some not. Work within your range of motion, with soft tissue work and our warm ups, your goblet squat will improve over time.

(33) Chest Press

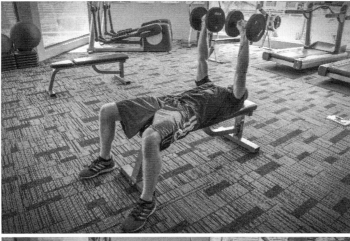

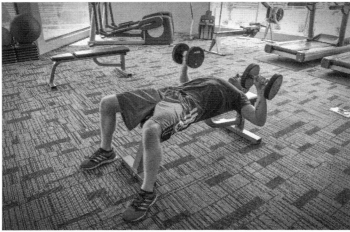

Strengthen your chest while also working the stabilizing muscles of the shoulder. This is the first variation I teach to my clients.

- Lie on a flat bench with a pair of dumbbells on your thighs.
- Use your thighs one at a time to lift the dumbbells above your chest.
- Arms extended, abs engaged, squeeze the dumbbells.
- Slowly lower the dumbbells to the outside of your chest until you get a 90-degree angle at your elbow.
- Contract your chest muscles by pushing the dumbbells back to the start position. A good tip is focus on getting your elbows closer to each other.

If new to this exercise please use a spotter, and practice getting the dumbbells into the start position.

(34) Cable Rows

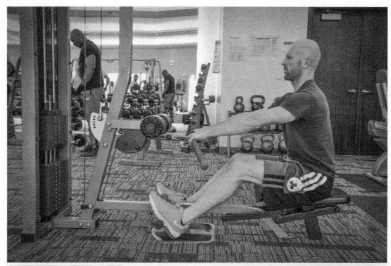

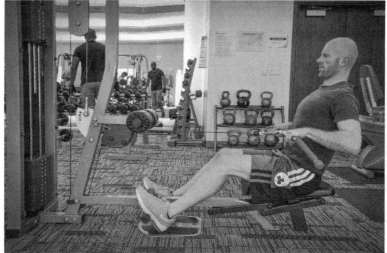

Good beginner horizontal row exercise. A good exercise to develop back strength without the risk of injuring your lower back.

- Sit on a low pulley machine and place feet on platform/bar, feet parallel and knees slightly bent.
- Lean forward and grab a straight bar.
- Keeping your back straight, lean back slightly and pull the bar to your belly button, keeping elbows close to your body.
- Focus on squeezing your shoulder blades together.
- Slowly return to start position.

(35) Lean and Press

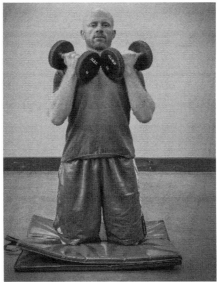

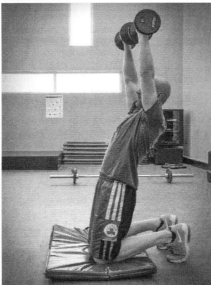

Great shoulder exercise while also working on your core and hamstrings.

- Tall kneel on a mat, knees hip distance apart and dumbbells shoulder height with palms facing your shoulders.
- Lean your shoulders and hips back slightly while engaging your glutes and core.
- Push the dumbbells overhead, extending the elbows and rotating the dumbbells 180 degrees, elbows should be pointing out in the top position.
- Return to start position.

(36) Plank

Level One

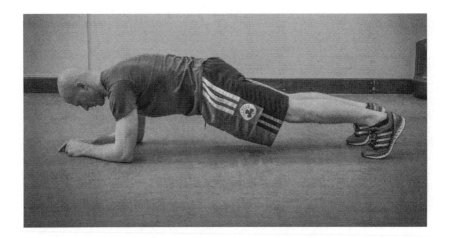

A safe core strengthening exercise and will help improve your posture.

- Get on all fours and place your elbows under your shoulders.
- Take your knees off the floor, brace your core and squeeze your glutes as hard as you can.
- Keep your back straight and your head in line with your spine.
- Do not let your hips drop below shoulder height.
- Controlled breathing throughout.

When 40 seconds become easy then progress to level two.

Level Two

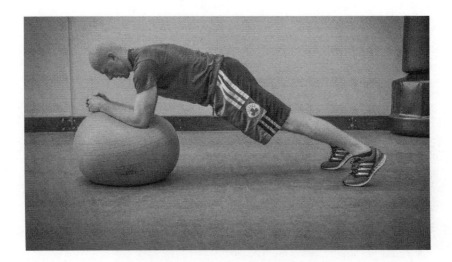

- With your knees on the floor, place your elbows on a fit ball, Elbows should remain under the shoulders throughout.
- Straighten one leg at a time, the wider your feet- the easier the exercise.
- Don't let your hips drop.
- Abs engaged and as always squeeze them glutes.

When you can do this for 40 seconds with feet together, then progress to level three.

Level Three

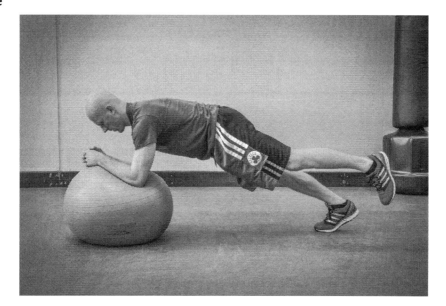

- Get into the same position as level two.
- Now, while keeping your hips in line with your elbows. Take one foot off the floor for five seconds and then repeat the opposite side.
- Try not to turn your hips, only your leg should move.
- Build up to 40 seconds.

(38) Mountain Climbers

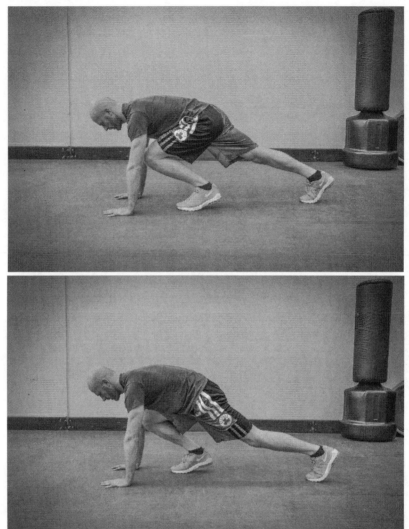

Awesome cardio with core and leg work thrown in. What's not to like? Oh yes, they are hell.

- Start in a push up position on a platform/floor.
- Maintain a straight line from ankles to your head.
- Lift your left knee to your chest and place foot on the floor under your hip.
- Then explosively switch feet, so your right knee is now close to your chest and left leg is extended.
- Repeat as fast as you can for time.

RECIPES

RECIPES

Over the years that I have been running the course, participants have been sending me recipes that include the foods I have listed. They found these on Pinterest and various sites. I have always told clients to go find recipes and to try new foods and ways of preparing food. By doing this you are always engaged in leading a healthy life. Going shopping and picking up certain ingredients for a recipe you will try later makes this program more enjoyable.

I have listed ten of the most popular recipes in this book just to give you a starting point. The meals are easy to make with basic ingredients. The ingredients can change depending on your tastes. Have fun in the kitchen and get used to preparing meals.

I recommend always making extra so you spend less time in the kitchen. Eating left over chicken and salad at work the next day will prevent you from getting the three cheese deluxe sandwich in Starbucks around the corner. Fail to prepare, prepare to fail.

Sometimes, for people like myself, you just want something quick and easy. Listen, throw some chicken breasts in aluminium foil, preheat oven to 450 and cook for twenty minutes. Then microwave some vegetables for a few minutes. That is a nutritious meal without much preparation that everyone can manage. It may not be fine dining, but it does the job.

Invest in some good Tupperware and use it every day. If you find it hard to cook during the week with your busy schedule, then prepare lots of meals on the weekend. Then just throw them in the microwave when you come home from work. All recipes I provided are easy to make.

Stick the food lists I provided on your fridge and get creative making meals from the list.

The recipes I included are:

- Steamed Broccoli with Balsamic Grilled Chicken
- Baked Salmon with Steamed Asparagus
- Shred Fat Omelette
- Spinach Leaf Salad with Pine Nuts
- Avocado Salad
- Sirloin Steak
- Sweet Potato Fries
- Oatmeal Bowl
- Banana Pancakes
- Oatmeal Power Balls

BALSAMIC GRILLED CHICKEN WITH STEAMED BROCCOLI
(Serves 4)

Ingredients:

- 4 boneless, skinless chicken breasts
- For Marinade:
- 1 cup balsamic vinegar
- ¼ cup dijon mustard
- ¼ cup olive oil
- 1 tbsp. all-purpose seasoning mix
- ½ tsp dried thyme
- ½ tsp garlic powder
- ½ tsp course ground pepper

Method:

Marinade

1. Mix all marinade ingredients into a jug.

Chicken

1. Trim all the fat and tendons from the chicken breasts.
2. Make small slits across each chicken breast to help the chicken cook more evenly and it will help the marinade stick to the chicken better.
3. Place the chicken in a plastic container or better yet a Ziploc bag. Lay them flat and pour in the marinade, then put in the fridge for at least 6 hours. This can be done early morning. Then when you come home from work you can begin grilling them.
4. When you're ready to cook, take the chicken out of the fridge and drain the bag of excess marinade. Leave the chicken to sit at room temperature while you preheat the grill. Oil a grill pan with non-stick grilling spray and turn the grill to medium-high.
5. When grill is hot, lay the chicken top side down diagonally across the grill grates and cook until you see grill marks, this will take approximately 3 minutes. As soon as you see marks, turn the chicken over and do the same for the other side for a few minutes.
6. When you have grill marks on both sides, turn the chicken and cook until it's browned on both sides. Cooking time will vary depending on the size of your chicken breasts, approximately 12-15 minutes for a 4-5ounce chicken breast.

Broccoli

1. Place broccoli in a steamer basket with a little water underneath and let steam for only 3-4 minutes so it doesn't lose to many nutrients.

Add some grass-fed butter to the broccoli and enjoy. This one takes a little preparation so, by preparing 4 chicken breasts you are sorted for tomorrow too.

BAKED SALMON WITH STEAMED ASPARAGUS
(Serves 1)

Ingredients:

- Fresh salmon fillet
- Asparagus
- Grass-fed butter
- Coarse salt and pepper
- Half a lemon

Method:

Salmon

1. Pre-heat oven to 450 degrees Fahrenheit (230 Celsius for the Irish).
2. Rinse Salmon in cold water, pat dry with paper towel.
3. Season the salmon with salt and pepper.
4. Place salmon skin side down on a non-stick baking sheet.
5. Bake until the salmon is cooked through, approximately 12 to 15 minutes.

Asparagus

1. Place in a steaming basket with a little water underneath for three minutes.

Serve with a teaspoon of grass-fed butter on the asparagus and a few drops of lemon juice. I love this simple recipe so much. It is a very popular one on the Reset Phase.

SHRED FAT OMELETTE
(Serves 1)

My favorite breakfast or late night snack. This only takes a few minutes to prepare and cook.

Ingredients:

- 3 medium eggs
- 1 garlic clove, minced
- 1 cup baby spinach, chopped
- 1 tbsp. of grass-fed butter
- Pinch of onion powder
- Pinch of sea salt
- Pinch of coarse black pepper
- Pinch of cumin

Method

1. In a bowl, beat 3 eggs and stir in the finely chopped baby spinach.
2. Season with the onion powder, salt, pepper and cumin.
3. Heat a small skillet on a stove and add the grass-fed butter.
4. When the butter melts add the garlic and stir until the garlic turns slightly brown.
5. Add the egg mix on top and let cook for about 3 minutes.
6. Flip with a spatula and cook for another 2 minutes.

Serve with some green leaves or half an avocado, or both. I really want you to be creative in the kitchen.

SPINACH LEAF SALAD WITH PINE NUTS
(Serves 4)

This is my favorite salad. It's quick and easy; just add some chicken.

Ingredients:

- 4 cups of baby spinach leaves
- 1 cup cherry tomatoes, sliced
- ¼ cup toasted pine nuts
- Splash of balsamic vinegar
- Splash of extra virgin olive oil

Season with:

- Coarse black pepper
- Sea salt
- Cayenne pepper

Method:

1. Heat a skillet on medium heat.
2. Add the pine nuts to the skillet for 5 minutes, stirring them occasionally. Watch them closely so they don't burn. Let them cool when time is up.
3. In a large salad bowl throw in the baby spinach, cherry tomatoes, pine nuts, balsamic vinegar and olive oil. Toss all the ingredients together and season with salt and pepper and serve with a protein of your choice.

If you have any balsamic chicken breasts, you can add one to this beauty of a salad.

AVOCADO SALAD
(Serves 3)

I love avocado. An avocado is full of healthy fats, and will help you feel full throughout the day. Serve this salad with chicken or an omelet and you will have an absolute powerhouse of a meal.

Ingredients:

- 1 ripe avocado- peeled, pitted and diced
- ½ onion- chopped
- ½ green bell pepper, chopped
- ½ large ripe tomato, chopped
- ½ lime, juiced
- Pinch of salt
- Pinch of pepper

Method:

1. Throw all ingredients in a salad bowl.
2. Mix all ingredients together and season with salt and pepper.

Boom, as easy as that!

SIRLOIN STEAK
(Serves 1)

Now, who doesn't love a good steak? This pan fried steak is delicious. Cook with coconut oil to get in some healthy fats into your body. Fish and chicken are my preferred protein choices, but I love a steak. Enjoy this one.

Cooking time: For medium cook for 2.5 minutes each side, for well-done cook for 4 minutes each side.

Ingredients:

- A grass-fed sirloin steak
- Coconut oil
- ¼ tsp sea salt
- ½ tsp black pepper
- Pinch of onion powder
- Pinch of garlic powder

Method:

1. To make the seasoning mix the sea salt, black pepper, onion powder and garlic powder together in a bowl.
2. Heat a cast iron pan on high heat for a few minutes.
3. Rub the steak with coconut oil on both sides and sprinkle the seasoning mix on both sides.
4. Once the pan is piping hot, add your steaks.

Serve it with some nice vegetables or salad. If this is your post workout meal in the Shred Phase, then add some amazing sweet potato fries.

SWEET POTATO FRIES
(Serves 4)

Sweet potato fries are super healthy, and in my opinion are better tasting than normal fries. Have these after a workout and share this little recipe with your friends and family. It's easy to prepare and I can bet you will make them more than once. It will make you want to workout knowing these babies await you when you come home.

Ingredients:

- 4 large sweet potatoes
- Olive oil
- Pinch of paprika
- Pinch of sea salt
- Pinch of garlic powder

Method:

1. Preheat oven to 450 degrees.
2. Wash and cut sweet potato into quarter inch thick long strips.
3. Line a baking tray with aluminum foil.
4. In a bowl toss the sweet potato in and cover with just enough olive oil to coat.
5. Sprinkle a little sea salt, paprika and garlic powder on and give them a shake.
6. Place the sweet potatoes on the foil, nicely spread out and put in oven to bake.
7. Bake for about 20-25 minutes, turning occasionally.

OATMEAL BOWL
(Serves 1)

The Oatmeal Bowl after a hard workout is exactly what your body needs. It is packed with protein, carbohydrates and fats. It is easy to make and should make you feel full. If you want, you can substitute the fruits listed for other fruits of your choice to add some variation.

Ingredients:

- 1 cup of water
- ½ cup oatmeal/ oat bran
- ¼ cup of raisins
- ¼ cup of raspberries
- 1 tbsp. almond butter
- 1 tbsp. hemp seeds
- 1 tbsp. chia seeds

Method:

1. In a saucepan, bring 1 cup of water to a boil.
2. Reduce the heat and add the oatmeal, blueberries and raspberries. Stir often to get your desired consistency.

3. Mix in the raisins, hemp seeds and chia seeds and stir.
4. Pour into a bowl and then add the almond butter to top.
5. Add extra water if desired.

BANANA PANCAKES
(Serves 1)

Quick, easy, low carb and delicious.

Ingredients:

- 2 eggs
- 1 Ripe medium banana

Method:

1. Using a fork, mash the banana in a bowl.
2. In a separate bowl, whisk the 2 eggs together.
3. Pour the eggs onto the banana and stir, until combined.
4. Heat a frying pan over medium heat, melt a little butter or coconut oil in the pan.
5. Drop about 2 tablespoons of the batter into the pan, fry each side for 30 seconds.

Serve with nuts, berries or a drop of honey.

OATMEAL POWER BALLS
(Many servings, depending on size)

The last recipe has to be something sweet. These Oatmeal Power Balls are packed with protein and healthy fats. They are a delicious treat after a grueling workout. They contain no refined sugars and are easily made in ten minutes.

The ingredients are not set in stone; you may replace the grass-fed butter with natural almond butter. You can add cinnamon or some dark chocolate squares if you like. Be creative and experiment. My daughter is a big fan of these, so much that I need to hide them at the back of the fridge.

Ingredients:

- 1 ½ cup rolled oats

- ½ cup protein powder (flavor of your choice)
- 6 soft dates, un-pitted
- ⅓ cup raisins
- Pinch of sea salt
- ½ cup grass-fed butter
- 1 tsp vanilla extract
- ½ cup coconut flakes

Method:

1. Add oatmeal, protein powder, grass-fed butter, 1 tsp vanilla extract, sea salt and un-pitted dates into a food processor and process until you have a sticky mixture.
2. Take out the sticky mixture and mix in the raisins.
3. Roll into balls using your hands.
4. Roll balls onto a plate of coconut flakes.
5. Store in fridge until ready to eat.

ABOUT THE AUTHOR

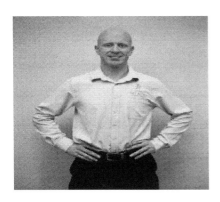

Robert Wilson is a coach, author, speaker and creator of the Shred Fat Program. Robert has helped many people lose unwanted body fat. Robert has been in the fitness industry for ten years and has been committed to educating people on safe exercise and on leading a healthy lifestyle.

Robert is a qualified personal trainer and strength and conditioning coach with ISSA. He has qualifications in corrective exercise, movement screening, anatomy and physiology, and lower back injury prevention and rehabilitation. He currently spends his time teaching, training, learning and writing in Saudi Arabia.